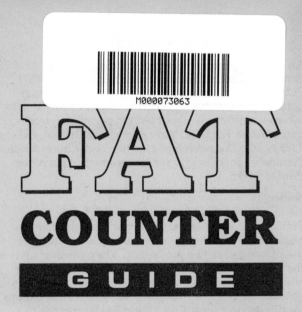

FAT
COUNTER
GUIDE

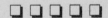

PUBLICATIONS INTERNATIONAL, LTD.

Notice:
Neither the Editors of Consumer Guide® and
Publications International, Ltd., nor the publisher take
responsibility for any possible consequences from the
use of material in this publication. The publisher advises
the reader to check with a physician before beginning
any dietary program or therapy. This publication does
not take the place of your physician's recommendations
for diet modification. Every effort has been made to
assure that the information in this publication is
accurate and current at the time of printing.

Editorial assistance: Donna Shryer

Contents

Introduction

WHY WORRY ABOUT FAT?

Your diet affects a lot more than just your waistline. Eating habits influence not only the shape of your body but your overall health as well.

Fat is a big part of the American diet. Fully 37 percent of the total calories we consume come from fat, most of which is saturated fat. Compared with many other countries, our consumption of saturated fat and cholesterol is unusually high. Although we need some fat in our diet for good health, too much of it can have the opposite effect.

One of the main reasons to adopt a low-fat diet is to combat coronary heart disease (CHD)—the formation of fatty deposits and blood clots on the walls of the coronary arteries, which supply blood to the heart muscle. Over time, a buildup of these deposits leads to a narrowing of the arteries. This causes a reduction in the flow of blood to the heart, just as stepping on a garden hose cuts down the flow of water to a lawn sprinkler.

Coronary heart disease is often called a silent killer because the deposits that clog the arteries build up gradually over the course of many years, often without giving any warning of what may lie ahead. Sometimes, the first symptom of CHD is a pain or an uncomfortable tightness, squeezing, or pressure of the chest, referred to as angina.

The heart is basically a muscle—an extraordinarily important and durable muscle, but like all muscles, one that requires nourishment to survive. And that nourishment is carried in the blood.

A heart attack occurs when the blood flow through a coronary artery to a portion of the heart is completely blocked and part of the heart muscle dies. If enough of the heart muscle is damaged, the victim may die. Unfortunately, for a large number of people, the first indication of CHD is the crushing pain from a serious and potentially fatal heart attack. The statistics tell the story: Heart attacks strike 1.25 million Americans each year, killing more than half a million of them. CHD is the leading cause of death in the United States.

Though it strikes many older people, CHD is not limited to the elderly. Nearly half of all heart attacks occur in people under the age of 65. What's more, the fatty deposits that may eventually block the arteries of adults can begin to form in childhood. CHD is not necessarily a part of growing older, however. You can take steps *now* to protect your own heart and to reduce the possibility of one day becoming a heart attack statistic.

While some of the factors that increase your risk of CHD are beyond your control—such as being male or having a family history of heart disease—there are three major risk factors you *can* control: cigarette smoking, high blood pressure, and a high level of cholesterol in the blood. If you smoke, you *can* stop. If you have high blood pressure, you *can* work with your doctor to get it under control. And if you have a high blood cholesterol level, you *can* make dietary changes to help reduce it. **Decreasing the amount of saturated fat in your diet is the most important way to reduce blood cholesterol levels.** That's one area where this *Fat Counter Guide* can help: It provides not only the values for fat and saturated fat, but it also gives percentages of calories from those two sources—a more useful and, in many ways, more accurate way to measure your dietary and saturated fat intake.

The benefits of a diet low in fat go well beyond reducing the risks of heart disease. The most common cancers found in this country, cancer of the breast, prostate, and colon, are also linked to high-fat diets.

For example, studies of various population groups show that people who eat a lot of fresh fruits and vegetables and consume whole-grain breads and cereals may receive protection from colon cancer because of the dietary fiber and vitamins these foods contain. But here again, fat in the diet has an impact. Perhaps most importantly, it affects bile, which the body produces to digest and absorb fat. The more fat there is in the diet, the more bile there will be available for delivery to the colon. Though some bile is necessary, too much of it may damage colon cells, possibly leading to tumors. There are, of course, many other factors, but the fat connection should not be overlooked.

It would be misleading to oversimplify a complex issue and imply that a low-fat diet will protect against these cancers. These are complicated diseases; much is unknown about them. The fundamental point is that a low-fat diet is clearly helpful in combating CHD, and it may have a beneficial influence with regard to cancer protection.

WHAT IS FAT?

Fat is nature's storehouse of energy-yielding fuel. Most fats are made up primarily of **triglycerides**—three fatty-acid chains attached to a glycerol molecule. To use the energy stored in fat, the body breaks down triglycerides into fatty acids. Individual cells then oxidize, or burn, the fatty acids for energy. Protein and carbohydrates such as sugars and starches also provide energy, but fat, with over two times the energy available per gram, is a denser fuel.

All living organisms, including plants, have the ability to manufacture fatty acids and assemble them into molecules of fat to store energy. Different species tend to manufacture different types of fat. As a general rule, animals manufacture a fat composed mainly of **saturated** fatty acids, and plants manufacture a fat that is rich in **polyunsaturated** fatty acids. Some plants also manufacture fat that contains a good deal of **monounsaturated** fatty acids, which are similar to polyunsaturated fatty acids but are much less complex.

Fats that consist primarily of saturated fatty acids are called **saturated fats**. They are typically solid at room temperature. Butter, lard, and the visible fat in meats are saturated fats. Much of the fat in milk (butterfat) is also saturated and solid at room temperature, but the process of homogenization breaks the fat into fine particles and scatters it throughout the liquid portion of the milk.

INTRODUCTION

On the other hand, **polyunsaturated fats** are usually liquid at room temperature. These liquid oils are found mostly in the seeds of plants. The oils from safflowers, sunflowers, corn, soybeans, and cotton are polyunsaturated fats made up primarily of polyunsaturated fatty acids.

Monounsaturated fats are also liquid at room temperature. Examples of fats rich in monounsaturated fatty acids are olive oil and canola (or rapeseed) oil. Avocados and nuts are also rich in this fat.

Sometimes vegetable oils are chemically modified to change some of their polyunsaturated fatty acids to saturated ones. This process, called **hydrogenation**, is useful commercially because it improves the shelf life of the oils and allows the less expensive vegetable oils to acquire important baking properties that are normally found in the more costly animal fats. **Hydrogenated** or **partially hydrogenated** vegetable oils are more saturated than the original oils from which they're made. Margarine and vegetable shortening are examples of such vegetable oils.

Although most animal fats are saturated and most vegetable fats unsaturated, there are some noteworthy exceptions. Fish and chicken fats have fewer saturated fatty acids and more polyunsaturated fatty acids than do red meats such as beef, veal, lamb, and pork.

By the same token, a few vegetable fats are so rich in saturated fats that they are solid at room temperature. Palm oil, coconut oil, and palm kernel oil contain between 50 and 80 percent saturated fat. Coconut oil and palm oil are widely used in the commercial production of nondairy creamers, snacks such as popcorn or chips, baked goods, and candy bars.

Foods rich in fat are usually those prepared by frying, basting, or marinating in butter, margarine, oil, or drippings from meats and poultry. Fat-rich foods can also be detected by their greasy textures. Sometimes fat can be seen as a solid whitish substance found around the perimeter of a cut of meat or running through it. In poultry, most of the fat comes from the skin. Dairy products such as whole milk, ice cream, whipped cream, and most cheeses are also rich sources of saturated fat. Commercially prepared baked goods such as pies, cakes, and cookies are common sources of hidden fats. Although we may think of them only as sweets, they are often prepared with hydrogenated oils that provide hefty doses of saturated fatty acids.

THE IMPORTANCE OF FAT
The energy your body uses comes from fuels in the foods you eat. (Carbohydrate and fat are the primary energy-yielding fuels, but under some limited circumstances protein can also be used for energy. Alcohol can be another fuel for the body.)

The amount of energy that can be obtained from a particular food is represented by the number of **calories** it produces when it is burned in the body. When you consume excess energy from food, that extra energy is stored in the body as fat.

Recent research suggests that if the extra energy is provided by carbohydrate, the body may step up its metabolism, and heat is produced. This is more likely to be the case if the person is physically active. In other words, if you exercise, you may be able to eat almost all the calories you want without worrying about excess body fat—as long as the calories come from carbohydrate. It is only when excess energy is consumed from fat and not from either carbohydrate or protein that this excess energy is likely to be stored as fat. (Alcohol is an exception, since sometimes energy consumed from alcohol can be stored as body fat.)

We all need some stored fat to provide our bodies with energy at times when we're not eating. Body fat is especially important as a source of energy during the night, because vital functions such as breathing and circulation require energy even while you're asleep. During pregnancy and childbirth, women acquire additional fat to support the fetus and to provide energy for the strain of labor and the production of milk after delivery.

Besides serving as stored energy, body fat has several practical purposes. A certain amount of fat in women is necessary to initiate and maintain menstruation. A cushion of fat distributed at strategic places throughout the body protects the heart, lungs, kidneys, and other organs from injury. And a layer of fat found just below the skin helps insulate us from heat loss.

The amount of fat in your body varies, depending on how much energy your body has stored. Only when an adult continually consumes more calories than the body needs for vital functions, daily activities, and exercise does body fat begin to accumulate, causing weight gain. Diabetes, high blood pressure, and heart disease are but a few of the health risks of being overweight.

WHAT IS CHOLESTEROL?

Cholesterol is a white, odorless, fatlike substance that is a basic component of the human body. In fact, each cell in the body is protected by a covering made up partly of cholesterol. Cholesterol is also used to make bile, a greenish fluid produced by the liver and stored in the gallbladder. The body needs bile to digest foods that contain fat and to absorb cholesterol from food. In addition, bile is needed to absorb vitamins A, D, E, and K (the fat-soluble vitamins).

Even though our bodies can make all the cholesterol we need, we also get it from many of the foods we eat. All animals produce cholesterol, and all foods that come from animal sources, such as meat, eggs, milk, cheese, and butter, contain cholesterol. Plants, on the other hand, do not manufacture cholesterol. All plant foods, such as cereals, grains, nuts, fruits, vegetables, and vegetable oils, contain no cholesterol.

CHOLESTEROL IN THE BLOOD

Some cholesterol is always present in the blood because the blood helps to transport cholesterol through the body. But cholesterol is one of a group of substances known as lipids (fats), which do not dissolve or mix with water. Blood happens to be made up of a substantial amount of water. Consequently, in order to move cholesterol through the bloodstream, the body wraps it in protein to form a molecule called a lipoprotein. The lipoproteins glide through the bloodstream carrying cholesterol through the body.

If cholesterol is normally present in your blood, why should you worry about it? The reason is that the total amount of blood cholesterol reveals how efficiently your body is using and managing its cholesterol. Excess cholesterol in the blood may mean that something is going wrong with the body's balancing mechanism.

Two types of lipoproteins play a major role in moving cholesterol through the blood. Low-density lipoproteins (LDLs) carry cholesterol to the body's cells, where it can be used in a variety of ways. In contrast, high-density lipoproteins (HDLs) are thought to carry cholesterol from the cells back to the liver so it can be absorbed in the bile and removed from the body.

When more of the cholesterol in your blood is carried by HDLs, there is less danger of an accumulation of cholesterol in the body. For that reason, HDLs are often referred to as "good" cholesterol. If, on the other hand, most of the cholesterol in your blood is carried by LDLs, there is an increased danger that cholesterol may accumulate in the body. The LDLs, which are often referred to as "bad" cholesterol, may take some of the unused cholesterol and deposit it on the walls of your coronary arteries. Over time, this buildup can begin to block the flow of blood to the heart, leading to a heart attack.

Periodic testing to measure the amount of cholesterol in the blood is important because such tests reveal how efficiently your body handles cholesterol. The most common test measures total cholesterol. Another test, lipoprotein analysis, determines how much of that cholesterol is in the form of HDLs and how much in LDLs.

WHAT CAUSES HIGH
BLOOD CHOLESTEROL?

The body has several mechanisms that enable it to balance the cholesterol it produces against what it obtains from food. When your diet provides a substantial amount of cholesterol, the body's output of cholesterol may be reduced. The body can also shed some excess cholesterol by using it to make bile and by dissolving some cholesterol in the bile that leaves the body through the feces.

In a very small minority of people (perhaps less than one percent of all those who have high blood cholesterol), an inherited defect can cause blood cholesterol levels to rise. This defect interferes with special receptor cells, located mainly on the surface of the liver, which are responsible for pulling cholesterol out of LDL molecules. When these receptors don't function properly, LDL cholesterol is stranded in the bloodstream.

For the vast majority of people whose blood cholesterol levels are too high, the major factor is not heredity. The problem is caused by diets that are high in total fat, saturated fat, and cholesterol.

HOW DIETARY FAT AFFECTS
BLOOD CHOLESTEROL

Not all sources of fat have the same impact on cholesterol. Saturated fat disturbs the body's cholesterol balance more than unsaturated fat does. For reasons that are not well understood, saturated fats suppress the production of LDL receptors, the ones responsible for pulling cholesterol out of the bloodstream. As a result, the total amount of cholesterol in the blood rises. Thus, **saturated fats in the diet tend to increase blood cholesterol.** In fact, no other dietary factor increases blood cholesterol as much as a high intake of saturated fat.

On the other hand, **polyunsaturated fats tend to lower total cholesterol levels** *when they replace saturated fats in the diet.* This is an important distinction to keep in mind. Adding large amounts of polyunsaturated fats to your diet without removing saturated fats will increase your total fat intake, and, as a consequence, your total calorie intake. Moreover, polyunsaturated fats are only half as effective at lowering cholesterol levels as saturated fats are at raising them. Another reason to eat polyunsaturated fats in moderation is that although such fats have the positive effect of lowering levels of LDL cholesterol, they may also lower the blood levels of the beneficial HDL cholesterol.

A diet high in monounsaturated fats from olive oil is believed to be responsible for the lower blood cholesterol levels found in people living in Mediterranean countries. The evidence indicates that **monounsaturated fats,** *when substituted for saturated fats in the diet,* **lower total blood cholesterol levels** by lowering LDL cholesterol levels without lowering HDL cholesterol levels.

The total amount of fat in your diet can also affect how your body deals with cholesterol, though its effect is less direct than the effect of saturated fat. A gram of fat provides more than twice as many calories as a gram of protein or carbohydrate. For that reason, a high-fat diet is likely to be a high-calorie diet as well. Any unneeded calories—those that are not burned off—are then stored in the body as fat. Over time, this will lead to weight gain and, eventually, obesity.

CHOLESTEROL IN THE DIET

Dietary cholesterol affects blood cholesterol levels by suppressing the production of LDL receptors. The impact of dietary cholesterol is less than that of saturated fat because of the body's feedback mechanism. This process slows the body's production of cholesterol when large amounts of it are consumed in the diet. But even if your body could adjust its cholesterol balance to accommodate a high-cholesterol diet, the large amount of saturated fat that usually accompanies cholesterol in food would once again upset the balance. The degree to which dietary cholesterol affects blood cholesterol levels seems to depend on how much total fat and saturated fat are eaten along with it.

The richest source of dietary cholesterol is egg yolks: A single egg yolk contains about 213 milligrams (mg) of cholesterol; as a component of the American diet, eggs contribute more than 35 percent of the total dietary cholesterol. Additional sources of cholesterol that are also rich in saturated fat and total fat include beef, pork, veal, lamb, whole milk, butter, cheese, cream, ice cream, sausages, frankfurters, and most luncheon meats.

IS YOUR BLOOD CHOLESTEROL LEVEL TOO HIGH?

The level of cholesterol in your blood is expressed in milligrams per deciliter (mg/dL), which indicates the amount of cholesterol found in one deciliter of blood. Research has shown that the risk of heart disease increases as the blood cholesterol level rises, especially as it climbs above 200 mg/dL. In the United States, adults who have a blood cholesterol level of 240 mg/dL or above appear to have more than twice the risk of developing CHD than those with readings below 200 mg/dL. Unfortunately, it has been estimated that more than 100 million Americans have a blood cholesterol level of 200 mg/dL or above—that's two out of every five people living in the United States.

Testing total blood cholesterol

To help you and your physician determine if your blood cholesterol level puts you at high risk for CHD, the National Cholesterol Education Program (NCEP) suggests that all adults aged 20 years or older have a cholesterol test. The NCEP also developed recommendations for classifying cholesterol levels and determining treatment. According to these guidelines, a total blood cholesterol level below 200 mg/dL is considered *desirable* for all adults aged 20 and older. A test result between 200 and 239 mg/dL is regarded as *borderline high,* whereas 240 mg/dL or more is rated as *high.*

If your blood cholesterol is in the desirable range, you should receive general information on your diet and risk factors and should be advised to have your cholesterol test repeated within five years. Verify all test results above 200 with a second test to confirm the results of the first test and to determine if further treatment is necessary.

If your test places you in the borderline-high range, you may need further evaluation with a different test, the lipoprotein analysis. This test is necessary only if you already have CHD or you have two or more additional risk factors:

- Being male
- Cigarette smoking
- High blood pressure
- Family history of premature (before the age of 55) CHD
- Low HDL cholesterol level (below 35 mg/dL)
- Advanced hardening of the arteries in the head, legs, feet, hands, or arms
- Severe obesity (30 percent or more over ideal bodyweight)

If your total blood cholesterol is in the borderline-high range, you do not have CHD, and you have fewer than two of the other risk factors for CHD, then you should receive information on the *Step One* diet, described in the next section. You should repeat the cholesterol test within one year.

In contrast, if your total blood cholesterol is in the borderline-high range and you have CHD or two or more risk factors for the disease, then you are advised to have an additional test—a lipoprotein analysis—within two months. Those who test in the high range should follow the same advice.

INTRODUCTION

Lipoprotein analysis

A lipoprotein analysis reveals how blood cholesterol is divided between LDL and HDL cholesterol. For an accurate result, this test must be performed twice. If the lipoprotein analysis reveals an LDL cholesterol level below 130 mg/dL, which is considered a desirable range, you should have your blood cholesterol tested again within five years.

If you have an LDL cholesterol level between 130 and 159 mg/dL (the borderline-high range), do not have CHD, and have fewer than two of the risk factors mentioned on page 17, then you should receive information on the *Step One* diet and have your cholesterol tested on a yearly basis.

The last category includes those who fall into the borderline-high group who do have CHD or two or more risk factors for CHD. Also in this category is the high-risk group, those who have lipoprotein test results of 160 mg/dL or more. Both groups should consider further evaluation by a physician to determine the causes of their high cholesterol.

DIETS TO LOWER BLOOD CHOLESTEROL

The *Step One* diet, recommended by the NCEP to lower blood cholesterol levels, restricts daily dietary cholesterol intake to less than 300 mg. Total fat is limited to 30 percent of calories, saturated fat to less than 10 percent. No more than 10 percent of total calories should come from polyunsaturated fats. Remaining fat calories in the daily diet should consist of monounsaturated fats.

If the *Step One* diet fails to lower your blood cholesterol to the desirable level, the *Step Two* diet may be recommended. The *Step Two* diet limits daily cholesterol intake to less than 200 mg and saturated fats to less than 7 percent of total calories. The portion of total fat allowed on this plan remains at less than 30 percent, since a diet that is much lower in fat would be difficult for most people to follow.

PUTTING YOUR DIET—AND THE COUNTER—TO WORK FOR YOU

The *Step One* diet, recommended to help reduce blood cholesterol levels for people in the borderline-high range, is actually the same heart-smart diet suggested for all adults, even those with normal cholesterol. It is also advised for children over the age of two. As a basic plan, it is designed to help you and your family eat a nutritious diet that is low in total fat, saturated fat, and cholesterol.

To adopt the *Step One* diet, you need to keep track of how much fat and cholesterol you consume each day. That may sound somewhat intimidating, but it doesn't have to be. By simply picking up this book, you've taken the important first step toward cleaning up your diet with a minimum amount of inconvenience.

The *Fat Counter Guide* lists the calorie, total fat, saturated fat, and cholesterol content of brand-name and common food items. It also gives the **percentage** of calories from each kind of fat. This way you can make wise food choices when you plan meals and shop for groceries.

Note that it isn't necessary to eliminate all foods from your diet that derive more than 30 percent of their calories from fat. When you do choose a meal that contains more than the recommended amount of fat, try to balance it out by making lower-fat choices the rest of the day. Keep in mind that you want your *overall* diet to provide less than 30 percent of your total calories from fat.

The same approach works with your intake of saturated fat: Use the values given in this counter for percentages from saturated fat; try to keep your intake within the recommended range of less than 10 percent of total calories for the *Step One* diet and less than 7 percent for *Step Two*.

The *Fat Counter Guide* also provides the cholesterol content for hundreds of individual food items. When planning meals, simply add up the cholesterol values shown to find out if the foods you plan to eat fit into your daily cholesterol "budget" of less than 300 mg (or less than 200 mg if you are on the *Step Two* diet). The counter makes it easy to compare similar foods.

AND CONSIDER THIS
Here are some additional tips to help you choose and prepare foods low in fat and cholesterol:

- Use low-fat dairy products, such as skim milk, low-fat cottage cheese, and nonfat yogurt.
- Eat poultry and fish more often than meat. When you do choose meat, select only lean cuts. Remove the skin from poultry, and trim away the visible fat from all meat before cooking.
- When buying canned tuna, salmon, or other fish, select products that are packed in water rather than oil.

- Try to limit your daily meat intake to no more than six ounces. Then fill the meals with low-fat foods like vegetables, pasta, and rice.
- Try venison, buffalo, and other wild game animals such as rabbit, pheasant, and duck; they generally contain less fat than domesticated animals bred for their meat.
- Avoid butter and margarine that is made from lard or shortening. As an alternative, use margarine that comes from polyunsaturated oils—corn, safflower, soybean, or sunflower.
- Include plenty of fruits in your diet; they contain no cholesterol and, except for avocados and olives, they are low in fat.
- When preparing meat, fish, or poultry, avoid frying. Bake, roast, or broil them instead. When basting, use wine, lemon juice, or tomato juice rather than fatty drippings.
- Avoid or decrease the consumption of processed luncheon meats and sausages, most of which are high in fat.
- Limit the use of peanut butter and peanut oil.
- Include cereals, breads, pasta, rice, and dried peas and beans frequently in your meals.
- Look for low-fat varieties of commercially prepared baked goods, such as pies and cakes, or prepare mixes at home with optional no-cholesterol recipes.
- Choose carefully at fast-food restaurants. Salads with low-fat dressing, plain baked potatoes, and broiled chicken without skin or sauce provide healthy alternatives to the usual fat-filled hamburgers and fries.

INTRODUCTION

THE FOOD GUIDE PYRAMID

A healthful diet is the cornerstone of any choles-terol-lowering program. Even in those cases where drugs are prescribed to reduce cholesterol, a diet low in saturated fat and cholesterol is still vital.

However, determining which foods fit into this low-fat, low-cholesterol diet can be difficult. That's why the U.S. Department of Agriculture

FOOD GUIDE PYRAMID

A Guide to Daily Food Choices

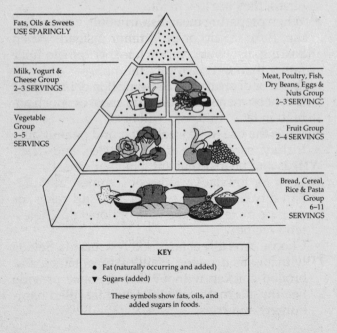

Fats, Oils & Sweets
USE SPARINGLY

Milk, Yogurt &
Cheese Group
2–3 SERVINGS

Meat, Poultry, Fish,
Dry Beans, Eggs &
Nuts Group
2–3 SERVINGS

Vegetable
Group
3–5
SERVINGS

Fruit Group
2–4 SERVINGS

Bread, Cereal,
Rice & Pasta
Group
6–11
SERVINGS

KEY

● Fat (naturally occurring and added)

▼ Sugars (added)

These symbols show fats, oils, and added sugars in foods.

developed the Food Guide Pyramid—to show generally what a healthful diet looks like.

The foundation of a healthful diet is complex carbohydrate, which should provide the bulk of your calories. Breads, cereals, pasta, and so on are low-fat and nutritious food choices. The second level contains the vegetable group and the fruit group; these foods are also virtually fat- and cholesterol free. The dairy group and the meat group (including legumes, nuts, and eggs) are near the top not because of their importance, but because they are to be a smaller proportion of the diet than the larger, lower levels. Finally, the tip of the pyramid represents the added sugar and fat in the diet; these should be used sparingly.

Using the Food Guide Pyramid to plan meals and snacks will help you stick to the *Step One* and even the *Step Two* diet. Let the number of daily servings per group be your guide. If your overall food choices generally have the same proportionality as the Pyramid, you will be on your way to a heart-healthy diet.

WHAT IS A SERVING?

Grain Group	1 slice of bread
	1 oz ready-to-eat cereal
	½ cup cooked cereal, rice, or pasta
Fruit Group	1 medium piece of raw fruit
	½ cup canned fruit
	¾ cup of fruit juice

INTRODUCTION

Vegetable Group	1 cup raw, leafy vegetables ½ cup cut-up vegetables ¾ cup vegetable juice
Meat, Poultry, Fish, Dry Beans, Eggs, and Nuts Group	2–3 oz cooked meat, poultry, or fish *May substitute for 1 oz meat:* ½ cup cooked dry beans 1 egg 2 tbsp peanut butter
Dairy Group:	1 cup milk or yogurt 1½ oz natural cheese 2 oz processed cheese

ABOUT THIS COUNTER

This fat counter provides values for hundreds of common foods, identified by brand or generic names, as well as about 200 items from fast-food menus. The data come from the U.S. Department of Agriculture, manufacturers and processors, and directly from food labels.

Separate columns list the calorie (CAL) and cholesterol (CHOL) content. Fat is broken down to show amounts of total (FAT) and saturated fat (SAT FAT). Fats are shown in grams (g); milligrams (mg) are used for cholesterol. Percentages of calories are included for both total and saturated fats to help those who follow the *Step One* and *Step Two* diets explained earlier.

With a simple formula, you can calculate the percentages for foods not included on our list:

Multiply grams of fat (or saturated fat) times 9, divide the result by the total number of calories, then multiply your answer by 100. This gives the percentage of total calories that come from fat (or saturated fat). For example, one raw egg contains 6 grams of fat and has 80 calories. Using the formula, multiply 6 by 9 to get 54; divide 54 by 80 to get 0.675; and multiply 0.675 by 100 to get 67.5 percent (rounded off to 68 percent). Thus, 68 percent of the calories in one raw egg comes from fat.

Foods on the list are grouped into common categories, such as "Beverages" and "Poultry," which are arranged in alphabetical order. After a brief description of each item, a specific portion size is given. The values in each column pertain to the portion size listed.

When trace amounts are shown for fat or saturated fat, it is impossible to calculate exact percentages, so "na" is used. However, as a practical matter, if only trace amounts of these elements are present, the percentage of calories they provide is generally quite low, usually less than 10 percent.

The symbol "<" means "less than," so "<1" indicates the presence of less than one unit of whatever is being measured (less than one percent, less than one gram). All of the fractional amounts have been rounded off.

Finally, while every effort has been made to ensure that the values listed are as accurate as possible, they are subject to change as food manufacturers modify the ingredients and methods of preparation.

Baked Goods

FOOD/PORTION SIZE	CAL.	FAT Total (g)	FAT As % of Cal.	SAT. FAT Total (g)	SAT. FAT As % of Cal.	CHOL. (mg)
CAKE						
Angel Food Cake Mix, Duncan Hines, 1/12 of cake (38 g)	130	0	0	0	0	0
Apple Cinnamon Snack Cake Mix, Sweet Rewards, Fat Free, Betty Crocker 1/8 pkg (44 g mix)	170	0	0	0	0	na
Chocolate, Snack Cake Mix, Sweet Rewards, Fat Free, Betty Crocker, 1/8 pkg (44 g)	170	0	0	0	0	na
Chocolate Loaf, Fat Free, Cholesterol Free, Entenmann's, 1/8 loaf (53 g)	130	0	0	0	0	0
Cupcakes Lights, Low Fat, Hostess, 1 cake (43 g)	140	1.5	10	0	0	0
Devil's Food Cake Mix, Moist Deluxe, Duncan Hines, 1/12 of cake, regular recipe (43 g)	290	15	47	3	9	45
Same as above, no-cholesterol recipe	280	15	48	2	6	0
Devil's Food Cake Mix, Super Moist, Betty Crocker 1/12 pkg (43 g)	270	4.5	15	1.5	5	0
Gingerbread, Mix, Dromedary, 1/8 pkg (70 g)	260	4	14	1	3	10
Lemon Snack Cake Mix, Sweet Rewards, Fat Free, Betty Crocker, 1/8 pkg (44 g mix)	170	0	0	0	0	na
Lemon Supreme Cake Mix, Moist Supreme, Duncan Hines, 1/12 pkg (43 g)	250	11	40	2	7	45
Same as above, no-cholesterol recipe	240	10	36	1.5	6	0
Pound Cake, All-Butter, Sara Lee, 1/4 cake (76 g)	320	16	45	9	25	85

FOOD/PORTION SIZE	CAL	FAT Total (g)	FAT As % of Cal	SAT FAT Total (g)	SAT FAT As % of Cal	CHOL (mg)
Pound Cake, Reduced Fat, Sara Lee, ¼ cake (76 g)	280	11	35	3	10	65
Twinkies Lights, Low Fat, Hostess, 1 cake (43 g)	130	1.5	10	0	0	0
White Cake Mix, Moist Deluxe, Duncan Hines, 1/12 of cake (43 g)	240	10	38	2	8	45
Same as above, no-cholesterol recipe	250	12	43	<3	<9	0
White Cake Mix, Moist Supreme, Pillsbury, 1/10 pkg (52 g)	220	5	20	1.5	6	0
White Cake Mix, Super Moist Light, Betty Crocker, 1/10 pkg (52 g mix)	210	3.5	15	1.5	6	0
Yellow Cake Mix, Super Moist, Light, Betty Crocker 1/10 pkg (52 g mix)	210	3	13	1.5	6	0
COFFEE CAKES & PASTRY						
Apple Strudel, Entenmann's, ¼ strudel	310	14	41	3.5	10	0
Apricot Danish Twist, Fat Free, Cholesterol Free, Entenmann's, ⅛ Danish	150	0	0	0	0	0
Black Forest Pastry, Fat Free, Cholesterol Free, Entenmann's, 1/9 Danish	130	0	0	0	0	49
Cheese Coffee Cake, Entenmann's, 1/9 cake	190	8	38	3.5	17	30
Cheese Filled Crumb Coffee Cake, Entenmann's, ⅛ cake	210	10	43	4	17	40
Cinnamon Apple Coffee Cake, Fat Free, Cholesterol Free, Entenmann's, 1/9 cake	130	0	0	0	0	0
Cinnamon Filbert Ring, Entenmann's, ⅙ Danish	270	17	57	3	10	30

BAKED GOODS

FOOD/PORTION SIZE	CAL	FAT Total (g)	FAT As % of Cal	SAT FAT Total (g)	SAT FAT As % of Cal	CHOL (mg)
Cinnamon Swirl Coffee Cake, Individual, Dolly Madison, 1 cake	170	6	32	2	11	15
Crumb Coffee Cake, Entenmann's, 1/10 cake	250	12	43	3	11	15
Crumb Coffee Cake, Sara Lee, 1/8 cake	220	9	3	1.5	6	15
Lemon Twist, Fat Free, Cholesterol Free, Entenmann's, 1/8 Danish	130	0	0	0	0	0
Pecan Danish Ring, Entenmann's, 1/8 Danish	230	15	59	3	12	25
Plain Coffee Cake, Dolly Madison, 2 cakes	270	11	37	3	10	15
Raspberry Cheese Pastry, Fat Free, Cholesterol Free, Entenmann's, 1/8 Danish	140	0	0	0	0	0
Raspberry Danish Twist, Entenmann's, 1/8 Danish	220	11	45	3	12	20
Walnut Danish Ring, Entenmann's, 1/8 Danish	230	14	55	3	12	25

COOKIES

FOOD/PORTION SIZE	CAL	FAT Total (g)	FAT As % of Cal	SAT FAT Total (g)	SAT FAT As % of Cal	CHOL (mg)
Chocolate Chip, Chips Ahoy, Nabisco, 3 cookies (32 g)	160	8	45	<3	<14	0
Chocolate Chip, Refrigerated, Pillsbury, 2 cookies, 1 oz (28g)	130	6	42	2	14	<5
Chocolate Sandwich, with Vanilla Creme, Reduced Fat, SnackWells, 2 cookies (26 g)	110	2.5	20	.5	4	0
Fig Newtons, Fat Free, Nabisco, 2 cookies (29 g)	100	0	0	0	0	0
Oatmeal Raisin, Fat & Cholesterol Free, Entenmann's, 2 cookies (24 g)	80	0	0	0	0	0

BAKED GOODS

FOOD/PORTION SIZE	CAL	FAT Total (g)	FAT As % of Cal	SAT FAT Total (g)	SAT FAT As % of Cal	CHOL (mg)
Oreos, Reduced Fat, Nabisco, 3 cookies (32 g)	140	5	32	1	6	0
Sugar Cookies, Refrigerated, Pillsbury, 2 cookies (32 g)	130	5	35	1.5	10	<5
Teddy Grahams, Graham Snacks, Cinnamon, Nabisco, 25 pieces (30 g)	140	4	26	1	6	0
Wafers, Sugar, Biscos, Nabisco, 8 cookies (28 g)	140	6	39	1.5	10	

PIE

FOOD/PORTION SIZE	CAL	FAT Total (g)	FAT As % of Cal	SAT FAT Total (g)	SAT FAT As % of Cal	CHOL (mg)
Apple, Entenmann's, 1/6 pie	300	14	42	3.5	11	0
Apple, Fat Free, Cholesterol Free, Entenmann's Beehive, 1/8 pie	270	0	0	0	0	0
Blueberry, 1/8 of 9-in. pie	360	17	43	4.5	11	0
Cherry, Fat Free, Cholesterol Free, Entenmann's, 1/5 pie	270	0	0	0	0	0
Chocolate creme, 1/8 of 9-in. pie	400	23	52	7	16	75
Coconut creme, 1/8 of 9-in. pie	430	23	48	8	17	85
Coconut custard, Entenmann's, 1/5 pie	340	19	50	8	21	135
Lemon, Entenmann's, 1/6 pie	340	17	45	4.5	12	45
Peach, 1/8 of 9-in. pie	460	19	37	5	10	<5
Pecan, 1/8 of 9-in. pie	500	27	49	5	9	110
Piecrust, Graham Cracker, Ready Crust, Keebler, 1/8 crust (21 g)	110	5	41	1	8	0
Pie Crust, Mix, Pillsbury 1/8 of 9-in. crust	100	6	54	1.5	5	0
Pumpkin, 1/8 of 9-in. pie	320	14	39	5	14	65

MISCELLANEOUS

FOOD/PORTION SIZE	CAL	FAT Total (g)	FAT As % of Cal	SAT FAT Total (g)	SAT FAT As % of Cal	CHOL (mg)
Brownie Mix, Blonde with White Chocolate Chunks, Blondies, Duncan Hines, 1/20 pkg (32 g)	170	8	42	2	11	15

BAKED GOODS

FOOD/PORTION SIZE	CAL.	FAT Total (g)	FAT As % of Cal.	SAT. FAT Total (g)	SAT. FAT As % of Cal.	CHOL. (mg)
Same as above, no-cholesterol recipe	170	7	37	2	11	0
Brownie Mix, Fudge, Betty Crocker, 1 brownie (34 g mix) as baked	200	9	41	2	9	25
Brownie Mix, Fudge, Low-Fat, Betty Crocker, 1 brownie (32 g mix)	130	2.5	17	.5	3	0
Doughnuts, Glazed, Buttermaid, 1 doughnut (44 g)	180	8	40	4	20	10
Doughnuts, Plain, Cinnamon or Powdered Sugar, Entenmann's 1 doughnut (52 g)	220	13	53	3	12	2
Pizza Crust, Original, Boboli, ⅛ shell (57 g)	160	3	17	1	6	5
Pizza Crust, Roll, Refrigerated, Pillsbury, ¼ pkg	180	2.5	13	.5	3	0

Baking Products & Condiments

FOOD/PORTION SIZE	CAL	FAT Total (g)	FAT As % of Cal	SAT FAT Total (g)	SAT FAT As % of Cal	CHOL (mg)
Bac'Os, Betty Crocker, 1 tbsp (7 g)	30	1	30	0	0	0
Baking Powder, Calumet, ¼ tsp (1 g)	0	0	0	0	0	0
Baking Soda, Natural, Arm & Hammer, ⅛ tsp (500 mg)	0	0	0	0	0	na
Barbecue Sauce, Original, Kraft, 2 tbsp (35 g)	50	0	0	0	0	0
Barbecue Sauce, Original, Open Pit, 2 tbsp (30 ml)	50	0	0	0	0	0

FOOD/PORTION SIZE	CAL	FAT		SAT FAT		CHOL (mg)
		Total (g)	As % of Cal	Total (g)	As % of Cal	
Barbecue Sauce, Thick & Tangy, Smoke House, Open Pit, 2 tbsp (30 ml)	50	0	0	0	0	0
Barley, Pearled, Brown's Best, ¼ cup dry (33 g)	100	0	0	0	0	0
Bulgur, uncooked, 1 cup	600	3	5	1	2	0
Butterscotch Topping, Smucker's, 2 tbsp (41 g)	130	0	0	0	0	0
Caramel Topping, Kraft, 2 tbsp (41 g)	120	0	0	0	0	0
Catsup, 1 tbsp	15	tr	na	tr	na	0
Chili powder, 1 tsp	10	tr	na	<1	na	0
Chocolate, Semi-Sweet, Baker's, ½ square (14 g)	70	4.5	58	2.5	32	0
Chocolate, Unsweetened ½ square (14 g)	70	7	90	4.5	58	0
Chocolate Chips, Real, Semi-Sweet, Baker's, ½ oz	60	3.5	53	2	30	0
Chocolate Chips, Semi-Sweet Morsels, Nestlé, 1 tbsp (14 g)	70	4	51	2	26	0
Chocolate Shell Topping, Hershey's, 2 tbsp (35 g)	230	18	70	7	27	0
Chocolate Topping, Dark, Dove, Smucker's, 2 tbsp (38 g)	140	5	32	1.5	10	0
Cinnamon, 1 tsp	5	tr	na	tr	na	0
Cocktail Sauce, Heinz, ¼ cup (60 g)	60	0	0	0	0	0
Cocoa Powder, Hershey's, 1 tbsp (5 g)	20	<1	<23	0	0	0
Coconut, Angel Flake, Sweetened, Baker's, 2 tbsp (15 g)	70	4.5	58	4	51	0
Coconut, Flakes, Sweetened, Peter Paul Mounds, 2 tbsp (15 g)	70	4.5	58	3.5	45	0
Cornmeal, degermed, enriched, dry, 1 cup	500	2	4	<1	na	0

BAKING PRODUCTS & CONDIMENTS

FOOD/PORTION SIZE	CAL	FAT Total (g)	FAT As % of Cal	SAT FAT Total (g)	SAT FAT As % of Cal	CHOL (mg)
Cornmeal, whole-ground, unbolted, dry, 1 cup	435	5	10	<1	na	0
Cornmeal, Yellow, Enriched-Degermed, Aunt Jemima, 3 tbsp (27 g)	90	.5	5	0	0	0
Cornmeal Mix, White, Self-Rising, with Flour, Salt and Baking Powder, Aunt Jemima, 3 tbsp (25g)	80	.5	5	0	0	0
Curry powder, 1 tsp	5	tr	na	na	na	0
Flour, All Purpose, Enriched, Bleached, Pillsbury Best ¼ cup (31 g)	110	0	0	0	0	0
Flour, All Purpose, Enriched, Unbleached, Pillsbury Best, ¼ cup (29 g)	100	0	0	0	0	0
Flour, Bread, Enriched, Pillsbury, ¼ cup (31 g)	110	0	0	0	0	0
Flour, buckwheat, light, sifted, 1 cup	340	1	3	<1	na	0
Flour, Self-Rising, Enriched, Bleached, Pre-Sifted, Pillsbury, ¼ cup (30 g)	100	0	0	0	0	0
Flour, Whole Wheat, Pillsbury, ¼ cup (33 g)	120	1	7	0	0	0
Frosting, Chocolate-Flavored, Creamy Deluxe, Betty Crocker, 2 tbsp (36 g)	150	6	36	1	6	0
Frosting, Chocolate Fudge, Frosting Supreme, Pillsbury, 2 tbsp (34 g)	140	6	39	<2	<10	0
Frosting, Vanilla, Creamy Homestyle, Duncan Hines, 2 tbsp (32 g)	140	5	32	1.5	10	0
Fruit Spread, All Flavors, Simply Fruit, Smucker's 1 tbsp (19 g)	40	0	0	0	0	0
Garlic powder, 1 tsp	10	tr	na	tr	na	0
Honey, Premium Clover, SueBee, 1 tbsp	60	0	0	0	0	0

FOOD/PORTION SIZE	CAL	FAT Total (g)	FAT As % of Cal	SAT FAT Total (g)	SAT FAT As % of Cal	CHOL (mg)
Horseradish, Prepared with Beets, Vita, 1 tsp (5 g)	0	0	0	0	0	0
Horseradish, Sauce, Kraft, 1 tsp (5 g)	20	<2	<68	0	0	<5
Hot Fudge, Light Topping, Smucker's, 2 tbsp (39 g)	90	0	0	0	0	0
Hot Fudge Topping, Kraft, 2 tbsp (41 g)	140	4	26	2	13	0
Jam, Concord Grape, Smucker's, 1 tbsp (20 g)	50	0	0	0	0	0
Jam, Strawberry, Smucker's Preserves, 1 tbsp (20 g)	50	0	0	0	0	0
Jelly, Concord Grape, Welch's, 1 tbsp (20 g)	50	0	0	0	0	0
Marshmallow Creme, Fluff, 2 tbsp (18 g)	60	0	0	0	0	0
Mayonnaise, Fat Free, Kraft Free, 1 tbsp (16 g)	10	0	0	0	0	0
Mayonnaise, Hellmann's, 1 tbsp (14 g)	100	11	99	<2	<14	5
Mayonnaise, Light, Reduced Calorie, Kraft, 1 tbsp (15 g)	50	5	90	1	10	5
Mayonnaise, Low Fat, Cholesterol Free, Hellmann's, 1 tbsp (17 g)	25	1	36	0	0	0
Mayonnaise, Real, Mayo, Kraft, 1 tbsp (14 g)	100	11	99	2	18	5
Molasses, Grandma's, 1 tbsp (15 ml)	50	0	0	0	0	0
Mustard, Dijon, Grey Poupon, 1 tsp (5 g)	5	0	0	0	0	0
Mustard, French's, Classic Yellow, 1 tsp (15 g)	0	0	0	0	0	0
Mustard, prepared yellow, 1 tsp or individual packet	5	tr	na	tr	na	0
Mustard, Spicy Brown, Grey Poupon, 1 tsp (5 g)	5	0	0	0	0	0
Onion powder, 1 tsp	5	tr	na	tr	na	0

BAKING PRODUCTS & CONDIMENTS

FOOD/PORTION SIZE	CAL	FAT Total (g)	FAT As % of Cal	SAT FAT Total (g)	SAT FAT As % of Cal	CHOL (mg)
Oregano, 1 tsp	5	tr	na	tr	na	0
Paprika, 1 tsp	6	tr	na	tr	na	0
Pepper, ground, black, 1 tsp	5	tr	na	tr	na	0
Picante Sauce, Medium, Pace, 2 tbsp (31.5 g)	10	0	0	0	0	0
Preserves, Apricot, Knott's Berry Farm, 1 tbsp (20 g)	50	0	0	0	0	0
Salad Dressing, Light, Miracle Whip, Kraft, 1 tbsp (16 g)	35	3	77	0	0	<5
Salad Dressing, Miracle Whip, Kraft, 1 tbsp (15 g)	70	7	90	1	13	5
Salsa, Mild, Medium or Hot, Thick & Chunky, Pace, 2 tbsp (30 ml)	10	0	0	0	0	0
Salt, Iodized, Morton, ¼ tsp (1.5 g)	0	0	0	0	0	0
Sandwich Spread, Kraft, 1 tbsp (15 g)	50	4	72	.5	9	<5
Seasoning Blend, Mrs. Dash, 1 tsp (1.3 g)	0	0	0	0	0	0
Seasoning Mixture, Original Recipe for Chicken, Shake 'N Bake, ¼ pouch	80	tr	na	tr	na	0
Shrimp Sauce, Hoffman House, 2 tbsp (30 g)	60	2	30	0	0	0
Soy Sauce, Kikkoman, 1 tbsp (15ml)	15	0	0	0	0	0
Soy Sauce, Milder, Kikkoman, 1 tbsp (15ml)	15	0	0	0	0	0
Soy sauce, ready to serve, 1 tbsp	11	0	0	0	0	0
Sugar, Brown, C & H 1 tbsp (4 g)	15	0	0	0	0	na
Sugar, brown, packed, 1 cup	820	0	0	0	0	0
Sugar, Confectioner's, 10x Powdered, Domino, ¼ cup (30 g)	120	0	0	0	0	0

FOOD/PORTION SIZE	CAL	FAT Total (g)	FAT As % of Cal	SAT FAT Total (g)	SAT FAT As % of Cal	CHOL (mg)
Sugar, powdered, sifted, spooned into cup, 1 cup	385	0	0	0	0	0
Sugar, white, granulated, 1 cup	770	0	0	0	0	0
Sugar, White, Pure Cane Granulated, Domino, 1 tbsp (4 g)	15	0	0	0	0	na
Sweet 'n Sour Sauce, Kraft Sauceworks, 2 tbsp (35 g)	60	0	0	0	0	0
Syrup, Chocolate, Hershey's, 2 tbsp (39 g)	100	0	0	0	0	0
Syrup, Chocolate, Lite, Hershey's, 2 tbsp (35 g)	50	0	0	0	0	0
Syrup, Lite, Log Cabin, ¼ cup (60 ml)	100	0	0	0	0	na
Syrup, molasses, cane, blackstrap, 2 tbsp	85	0	0	0	0	0
Syrup, Natural Apricot, Smucker's, (and all natural "fruit" flavors) ¼ cup (60 ml)	210	0	0	0	0	0
Syrup, Regular, Log Cabin, ¼ cup (59 ml)	200	0	0	0	0	0
Tabasco Sauce, 1 tsp (5 g)	0	0	0	0	0	0
Tartar Sauce, Fat Free, Cholesterol Free, Nonfat, Kraft, 2 tbsp (32 g)	25	0	0	0	0	0
Tartar Sauce, Hellmann's, 2 tbsp (28 g)	140	16	100	2.5	16	10
Tartar Sauce, Hoffman House, 2 tbsp (30 g)	130	12	83	2	14	na
Vinegar, Apple Cider, Heinz, ½ fl oz	2	0	0	0	0	0
Vinegar, Distilled White, Heinz, ½ fl oz	2	0	0	0	0	0
Vinegar, Red or White Wine, Regina, 2 tbsp (15ml)	0	0	0	0	0	0
Worcestershire Sauce, Lea & Perrins, 1 tsp (5 g)	5	0	0	0	0	na

BAKING PRODUCTS & CONDIMENTS

FOOD/PORTION SIZE	CAL	FAT Total (g)	FAT As % of Cal	SAT FAT Total (g)	SAT FAT As % of Cal	CHOL (mg)
Yeast, Active Dry, Fleischmann's, ¼ tsp per bread slice	0	0	0	0	0	0
Yeast, baker's dry active, 1 pkg	20	tr	na	tr	na	0
Yeast, brewer's dry, 1 tbsp	25	tr	na	tr	na	0
Yeast, RapidRise, Fleischmann's, ¼ tsp per bread slice	0	0	0	0	0	0

Beverages

ALCOHOL						
Beer, light, 12 fl oz	95	0	0	0	0	0
Beer, regular, 12 fl oz	150	0	0	0	0	0
Gin, rum, vodka, whiskey, 80 proof, 1½ fl oz	97	0	0	0	0	0
Gin, rum, vodka, whiskey, 90 proof, 1½ fl oz	110	0	0	0	0	0
Wine, table, red, 3½ fl oz	74	0	0	0	0	0
Wine, table, white, 3½ fl oz	70	0	0	0	0	0

COFFEE						
Cafe Francais, General Foods International Coffees, 8 fl oz, 1⅓ tbsp mix	60	3.5	53	1	15	0
Coffee Flavor Instant Hot Beverage, Postum, 8 fl oz, 1 tsp mix	10	0	0	0	0	0
Instant, Folger's, 6 fl oz, 1 tsp mix	0	0	0	0	0	0
Instant, French Vanilla, Taster's Choice, 8 fl oz, 1 tsp mix	5	0	0	0	0	0

FOOD/PORTION SIZE	CAL	FAT Total (g)	FAT As % of Cal	SAT FAT Total (g)	SAT FAT As % of Cal	CHOL (mg)
Regular, all grind varieties, 100% coffee, unlimited	0	0	0	0	0	0
Swiss Mocha, Sugar Free, General Foods International Coffees, 8 fl oz, 1⅓ tbsp mix	30	2	60	.5	15	0
JUICE						
Apple, bottled, Musselman's, 8 fl oz	120	0	0	0	0	0
Apple, Pure 100%, Mott's, 8 fl oz (240 ml)	120	0	0	0	0	0
Apple Strawberry Banana, from Concentrate, Apple Quenchers, Juice Cocktail, Very Fine, 8 fl oz (240 ml)	120	0	0	0	0	0
Black Cherry White Grape, Boku, 1½ cup (355 ml)	180	0	0	0	0	0
Cherry, Bottled, from Concentrate, Orchards Best, Minute Maid, 8 fl oz (240 ml)	110	0	0	0	0	0
Cherry, with Other Natural Flavors, Canned, from Concentrate, Juicy Juice, Libby's, 8 fl oz (240 ml)	140	0	0	0	0	0
Cranapple, Bottled, from Concentrate, Ocean Spray, 8 fl oz (240 ml)	160	0	0	0	0	0
Cranberry Juice Cocktail, Ocean Spray, 8 fl oz (240 ml)	140	0	0	0	0	0
Grape, Bottled, from Concentrate, Welch's 8 fl oz (240 ml)	170	0	0	0	0	0
Grape, Frozen Concentrate, Welch's, 8 fl oz	160	0	0	0	0	0
Grape, Juice Cocktail, Light, Welch's, 8 fl oz	50	0	0	0	0	0

BEVERAGES

FOOD/PORTION SIZE	CAL	FAT Total (g)	FAT As % of Cal	SAT FAT Total (g)	SAT FAT As % of Cal	CHOL (mg)
Grapefruit, Bottled, from Concentrate, Ocean Spray, 8 fl oz (240 ml)	100	0	0	0	0	0
Grapefruit, raw, 1 cup	95	tr	na	tr	na	0
Grapefruit, Ruby Red, Bottled, from Concentrate, Very Fine, 8 fl oz (240 ml)	120	0	0	0	0	0
Grapefruit, Ruby Red & Tangerine, Bottled, from Concentrate, Ocean Spray, 8 fl oz (240 ml)	130	0	0	0	0	0
Island Guava, Bottled, from Concentrate, Ocean Spray, 8 fl oz (240 ml)	130	0	0	0	0	0
Lemon, raw, 1 cup	60	tr	na	tr	na	0
Lemon, ReaLemon Juice, from Concentrate, Borden, 1 tsp (5 ml)	0	0	0	0	0	0
Lemonade, Frozen Concentrate, Minute Maid, 8 fl oz	110	0	0	0	0	0
Lemon-Lime, Gatorade, 8 fl oz (240 ml)	50	0	0	0	0	0
Lime, Bottled, from Concentrate, ReaLime, 1 tsp (5 ml)	0	0	0	0	0	0
Lime, raw, 1 cup	65	tr	na	tr	na	0
Orange, Bottled, from Concentrate, Very Fine, 10 fl oz (296 ml)	130	0	0	0	0	0
Orange, from Concentrate, Chilled, Season's Best, Tropicana, 8 fl oz	110	0	0	0	0	0
Orange, Frozen Concentrate, Minute Maid, 8 fl oz	110	0	0	0	0	0
Orange, Not from Concentrate, Chilled, Pure Premium, Tropicana, 8 fl oz	110	0	0	0	0	0
Orange, raw, 1 cup	110	tr	na	<1	<1	0

FOOD/PORTION SIZE	CAL	FAT Total (g)	FAT As % of Cal	SAT FAT Total (g)	SAT FAT As % of Cal	CHOL (mg)
Orange Cranberry, Bottled, from Concentrate, Twister, Tropicana, 8 fl oz (240 ml)	130	0	0	0	0	0
Peach, Orchard Peach, Dole, 8 fl oz (240 ml)	140	0	0	0	0	0
Pear, Canned, from Concentrate, Libby's, 11.5 fl oz (340 ml)	220	0	0	0	0	0
Pineapple, Canned, Unsweetened, Not from Concentrate, Dole, 8 fl oz (240 ml)	110	0	0	0	0	0
Prune, Sunsweet, 8 fl oz (240 ml)	180	0	0	0	0	0
Tomato, Bottled, from Concentrate, Campbell's, 8 fl oz (240 ml)	50	0	0	0	0	0
Tropical Blend, Unfrozen Concentrate, Mott's In-A-Minute, 8 fl oz	130	0	0	0	0	0
Tropical Orange Passion, Pourable Concentrate, Juice Maker's, Welch's, 8 fl oz	140	0	0	0	0	0
Vegetable Juice, V-8, 8 fl oz (240 ml)	50	0	0	0	0	0
MILK						
Buttermilk, 1 cup	100	2	18	1	9	9
Buttermilk, Cultured, Lowfat (1 1/2%), Dean's, 1 cup (240 ml)	120	3.5	26	2.5	19	20
Canned, Condensed, Sweetened, Carnation, 2 tbsp (30 ml)	130	3	21	2	14	10
Canned, Evaporated, Skim, Milnot, 2 tbsp (30 ml)	25	0	0	0	0	0
Canned, Evaporated, Whole, Pet, 2 tbsp	40	2	45	1	23	5

BEVERAGES

FOOD/PORTION SIZE	CAL	FAT Total (g)	FAT As % of Cal	SAT FAT Total (g)	SAT FAT As % of Cal	CHOL (mg)
Chocolate, low fat (1%), 1 cup	160	3	17	2	11	7
Chocolate, low fat (2%), 1 cup	180	5	25	3	15	17
Chocolate Malt Flavor, Ovaltine Classic, ¾ oz	80	0	0	0	0	0
Cocoa Mix, Milk Chocolate, Carnation, 1 envelope	110	1	8	tr	na	1
Cocoa Mix, Rich Chocolate, Carnation, 1 envelope	110	1	8	1	8	1
Dried, nonfat, instant, Sanalac, ¼ cup (24 g)	90	0	0	0	0	0
Eggnog (commercial), 1 cup	340	19	50	11	29	149
Evaporated Filled Milk, Milnot, 2 tbsp (30 ml)	40	2	45	0	0	0
Evaporated Skim Milk, Lite, Carnation, 2 tbsp	25	0	0	0	0	3
Lowfat (2%), Dean's, 1 cup	130	5	35	3	21	20
Low fat (2%), milk solids added, 1 cup	125	5	36	3	22	18
Low fat (2%), no milk solids, 1 cup	120	5	38	3	23	18
Malted, chocolate, powder, ¾ oz	84	1	11	<1	<5	1
Malted, chocolate, powder, prepared with 8 oz whole milk	235	9	34	6	23	34
Malted, Chocolate, Prepared, Dean's, ½ pint (236 ml)	330	9	25	6	16	40
Nonfat (Skim), Dean's, 1 cup (240 ml)	90	0	0	0	0	<5
Nonfat (skim), milk solids added, 1 cup	90	1	10	<1	<4	5
Nonfat (skim), no milk solids, 1 cup	85	tr	na	<1	<3	4
Quik, Chocolate, Nestlé, 2 tbsp (22 g)	90	<1	<5	<1	<5	0
Whole (3.3% fat), 1 cup	150	8	48	5	30	33

CONSUMER GUIDE®

FOOD/PORTION SIZE	CAL	FAT		SAT FAT		CHOL (mg)
		Total (g)	As % of Cal	Total (g)	As % of Cal	
SOFT DRINKS, CARBONATED						
Club Soda, Schweppes, 8 fl oz (240 ml)	0	0	0	0	0	0
Coca-Cola Classic, 1 can	140	0	0	0	0	0
Diet Coke, 1 can	0	0	0	0	0	0
Diet Coke, Caffeine Free, 1 can	0	0	0	0	0	0
Diet Dr. Pepper, 1 can	0	0	0	0	0	0
Diet Pepsi, 1 can	0	0	0	0	0	0
Diet Pepsi, Caffeine Free, 1 can	0	0	0	0	0	0
Diet-Rite, Cola, 1 can	0	0	0	0	0	0
Diet-Rite, Red Raspberry, 1 can	0	0	0	0	0	0
Fresca, 1 can	0	0	0	0	0	0
Ginger Ale, Schweppes, 8 fl oz (240 ml)	90	0	0	0	0	0
Grape, Carbonated, Crush, 1 can	210	0	0	0	0	0
Orange, Carbonated, Crush, 1 can	210	0	0	0	0	0
Pepsi-Cola, Caffeine-Free, 1 can	150	0	0	0	0	0
Root Beer, Dad's, 1 can (12 oz)	165	0	0	0	0	0
Root Beer, Dad's, Diet, 1 can	0	0	0	0	0	0
7-Up, 1 can	140	0	0	0	0	0
7-Up, Diet, 1 can	0	0	0	0	0	0
SOFT DRINKS, NONCARBONATED						
Country Time Drink Mix, Sugar Sweetened, Lemonade/Pink Lemonade, mix for 8 fl oz (18 g)	70	0	0	0	0	0

BEVERAGES

FOOD/PORTION SIZE	CAL	FAT Total (g)	FAT As % of Cal	SAT FAT Total (g)	SAT FAT As % of Cal	CHOL (mg)
Country Time Sugar Free Drink Mix, Lemonade/Pink Lemonade, ⅛ tub, 8 fl oz (1.9 g)	5	0	0	0	0	0
Country Time Sugar Free Drink Mix, Lemon-Lime, ⅛ tub, 8 fl oz (1.9 g)	5	0	0	0	0	0
Crystal Light Sugar Free Drink Mix, all flavors, 8 fl oz (1.7 g)	5	0	0	0	0	0
Grape Drink, Juice Box, Juicy Juice, 1 box	80	0	0	0	0	0
Grape drink, noncarbonated, canned, 6 fl oz	100	0	0	0	0	0
Hawaiin Punch, Tidal Wave Tropical Fruit, Typhoon Blasters, 1 box (250 ml)	130	0	0	0	0	0
Hi-C Drink, Boppin' Berry, 8 fl oz	130	0	0	0	0	0
Hi-C Drink, Ecto Cooler, 8 fl oz	130	0	0	0	0	0
Hi-C Drink, Grape, 8 fl oz	130	0	0	0	0	0
Hi-C Drink, Hula Punch, 8 fl oz	120	0	0	0	0	0
Hi-C Drink, Orange, 8 fl oz	120	0	0	0	0	0
Kool-Aid Soft Drink Mix, Unsweetened, all flavors, 8 fl oz (0.6 g)	0	0	0	0	0	0
Kool-Aid Sugar-Free Soft Drink Mix, all flavors, 8 fl oz (1.1 g)	5	0	0	0	0	0
Lemonade Concentrate, Frozen, Diluted, Minute Maid, 8 fl oz	110	0	0	0	0	0
Ocean Spray, Cran-Apple Drink, 8 fl oz (240 ml)	160	0	0	0	0	0
Ocean Spray, Cran-Grape Drink, 8 fl oz (240 ml)	150	0	0	0	0	0

FOOD/PORTION SIZE	CAL	FAT Total (g)	FAT As % of Cal	SAT FAT Total (g)	SAT FAT As % of Cal	CHOL (mg)
Ocean Spray, Cran-Raspberry Drink, 8 fl oz (240 ml)	140	0	0	0	0	0
Pineapple-grapefruit juice drink, 6 fl oz	90	tr	na	0	0	0
Wyler's Punch Mix, Unsweetened, all flavors, 8 fl oz (0.6 g)	0	0	0	0	0	0
TEA						
Brewed, Lipton, 1 tea bag	0	0	0	0	0	0
Iced Tea, Sugar Free, Drink Mix, Crystal Light, 8 fl oz (1.1 g)	5	0	0	0	0	0
Instant, powder, sweetened, 8 fl oz	85	tr	na	tr	na	0
Instant, powder, unsweetened, 8 fl oz	tr	tr	na	tr	na	0
Instant, Sugar Sweetened, Natural Brew, Lipton 1⅔ tbsp for 8 oz prepared	90	0	0	0	0	0
Instant, Unsweetened, Lipton, 1½ tsp	0	0	0	0	0	0

Breads & Cereals

FOOD/PORTION SIZE	CAL	FAT Total (g)	FAT As % of Cal	SAT FAT Total (g)	SAT FAT As % of Cal	CHOL (mg)
BISCUITS						
Baking powder, Mix, Bisquick, ⅓ cup mix	170	6	32	1.5	8	0
Buttermilk, Mix, Jiffy, ⅓ cup mix	160	4	23	2	11	<5
Buttermilk, Refrigerated, Pillsbury, 3 biscuits	150	2	12	0	0	0

BREADS & CEREALS

FOOD/PORTION SIZE	CAL	FAT Total (g)	FAT As % of Cal	SAT FAT Total (g)	SAT FAT As % of Cal	CHOL (mg)
BREAD						
Boston brown, canned, 3¼ x ¼-in. slice	95	1	9	<1	<3	3
Cracked-wheat, 1 slice	65	1	14	<1	<3	0
Crumbs, enriched, dry, grated, 1 cup	390	5	12	2	5	5
Crumbs, French Style, Gonnella, ¼ cup (28 g)	110	1.5	12	0	0	0
French, enriched, 5 x 2½ x 1-in. slice	100	1	9	<1	<3	0
French, Enriched, Gonnella, 1 slice (28 g)	80	1	11	0	0	0
Frozen Bread Dough, Texas White Roll, Rhodes, 1 roll (56.7 g)	150	3	18	0	0	0
Frozen, White Bread Dough, Rhodes, 1 slice (50 g)	140	2	13	0	0	0
Italian, enriched, 4½ x 3¼ x ¾-in. slice	85	tr	na	tr	na	0
Italian, Hearth Baked, Gonnella, 2 slices (36 g)	90	1.5	15	0	0	0
Oat, Hearty Slices Crunchy Oat Bread, Pepperidge Farm, 1 slice, 1.4 oz (38 g)	100	2	18	0	0	0
Oat Bran, Roman Meal, 1 slice (28 g)	70	1	13	0	0	0
Pita, enriched, white, 6-in. diameter, 1 pita	165	1	5	<1	<1	0
Pita, White, Sahara, Thomas', 1 pita (57 g)	150	1	6	0	0	0
Pumpernickel Rye, Natural, Brownberry, 1 slice (28 g)	70	.5	6	0	0	0
Raisin, Cinnamon Swirl, Pepperidge Farm, 1 slice (28 g)	80	1.5	17	0	0	0
Raisin, enriched, 1 slice	65	1	14	<1	<3	0

FOOD/PORTION SIZE	CAL	FAT Total (g)	FAT As % of Cal	SAT FAT Total (g)	SAT FAT As % of Cal	CHOL (mg)
Rye, Bohemian Style, S. Rosen's, 1 slice (38 g)	90	1	10	0	0	0
Rye, ⅔ wheat, ⅓ rye, 4¾ x 3¾ x ⁷⁄₁₆-in. slice	65	1	14	<1	<3	0
Vienna, enriched, 4¾ x 4 x ½-in. slice	70	1	13	<1	<3	0
Vienna, Old Fashioned, Turano, 2 slices (38 g)	90	.5	5	0	0	0
Wheat, Natural, Brownberry, 1 slice (36 g)	80	1	11	0	0	0
Wheat, Soft, Brownberry, 1 slice (32 g)	80	2	23	0	0	0
Wheat, Stone Ground, Country Hearth, 1 slice (42 g)	90	.5	5	0	0	0
White, Country White Hearty Slices, Pepperidge Farm, 1 slice, 1.4 oz (38 g)	90	1	10	0	0	0
White, Home Pride Buttertop, 1 slice (27 g)	70	1	13	0	0	0
White, Regular, Wonder, 2 slices (43 g)	100	1.5	14	0	0	0
Whole-wheat, 16-slice loaf, 1 slice	70	1	13	<1	<5	0
Whole Wheat, Roman Meal, 1 slice (28 g)	60	1	15	0	0	0

CEREALS, COLD

FOOD/PORTION SIZE	CAL	FAT Total (g)	FAT As % of Cal	SAT FAT Total (g)	SAT FAT As % of Cal	CHOL (mg)
All-Bran, Kellogg's, ½ cup, 1.1 oz (30 g)	80	1	11	0	0	0
Alpha-Bits, Post, 1 cup (32 g)	130	1.5	10	0	0	0
Apple Jacks, Kellogg's, 1 cup, 1.1 oz (30 g)	110	0	0	0	0	0
Bran Flakes, Post, 1 cup (51 g)	200	3	14	.5	2	0
Cap'n Crunch, Quaker, ¾ cup (27 g)	110	1.5	12	.5	4	0

BREADS & CEREALS

FOOD/PORTION SIZE	CAL	FAT Total (g)	FAT As % of Cal	SAT FAT Total (g)	SAT FAT As % of Cal	CHOL (mg)
Cap'n Crunch's Peanut Butter Crunch, Quaker, ¾ cup (27 g)	110	2.5	20	.5	4	0
Cheerios, General Mills, 1 cup (30 g)	110	2	16	0	0	0
Cheerios, Honey-Nut, General Mills, 1 cup (30 g)	120	<2	<11	0	0	0
Cocoa Krispies, Kellogg's, ¾ cup (31 g)	120	1	8	.5	4	0
Cocoa Pebbles, Post, ¾ cup (29 g)	120	1	8	1	8	0
Cocoa Puffs, General Mills, 1 cup (30 g)	120	1	8	0	0	0
Common Sense Oat Bran, Kellogg's, ¾ cup, 1.1 oz (30 g)	110	1	8	0	0	0
Complete Bran Flakes, Kellogg's, ¾ cup (29 g)	90	.5	5	0	0	0
Corn Chex, Ralston Purina, 1¼ cups (30 g)	110	0	0	0	0	0
Corn Flakes, Kellogg's, 1 cup, 1 oz (28 g)	100	0	0	0	0	0
Corn Flakes, Total, 1⅓ cup (30 g)	110	.5	4	0	0	0
Cracklin' Oat Bran, Kellogg's, ¾ cup, 2 oz (55 g)	230	8	31	3	12	0
Frosted Flakes, Kellogg's, ¾ cup, 1.1 oz (30 g)	120	0	0	0	0	0
Frosted Mini-Wheats, Bite Size, Kellogg's, 1 cup (59 g)	200	1	5	0	0	0
Fruit & Fibre–Dates, Raisins, Walnuts, Post, 1 cup (51 g)	200	3	14	.5	2	0
Fruit Loops, Kellogg's, 1 cup (32 g)	130	1	7	.5	3	0
Fruity Pebbles, Post, ¾ cup (27 g)	110	1	8	<1	<4	0

FOOD/PORTION SIZE	CAL	FAT		SAT FAT		CHOL
		Total (g)	As % of Cal	Total (g)	As % of Cal	(mg)
Golden Grahams, General Mills, ¾ cup (30 g)	120	1	8	0	0	0
Granola, Fruit, Low Fat, Nature Valley, General Mills, ⅔ cup (55 g)	210	2.5	11	0	0	0
Grape-Nuts, Post, ½ cup (58 g)	200	0	0	0	0	0
Grape-Nuts Flakes, Post, ¾ cup (29 g)	100	1	9	0	0	0
Honeycomb, Post, 1⅓ cups (29 g)	110	0	0	0	0	0
Just Right with Fiber Nuggets, Kellogg's, 1 cup (55 g)	210	<2	<9	0	0	0
Just Right with Fruit & Nuts, Kellogg's, 1 cup (55 g)	200	2	9	0	0	0
Kix, General Mills, 1⅓ cups (30 g)	120	.5	0	0	0	0
Life, Cinnamon, Quaker Oats, ¾ cup (50 g)	120	1	8	0	0	0
Life, Quaker Oats, ¾ cup (32 g)	120	<2	<11	0	0	0
Lucky Charms, General Mills, 1 cup (30 g)	120	1	8	0	0	0
Multi-Grain Squares, Healthy Choice, Kellogg's, 1¼ cups (55 g)	190	1	5	0	0	0
Nutri-Grain Almonds & Raisins, Kellogg's, 1¼ cups (49 g)	180	3	15	0	0	0
Nutri-Grain, Golden Wheat, Kellogg's, ¾ cup (30 g)	100	1	9	0	0	0
Oat Bran, Quaker, 1¼ cups (57 g)	210	3	13	<1	<2	0
100% Bran, Nabisco/Post, ⅓ cup	80	.5	6	0	0	0
100% Natural, Granola, Oats & Honey, Quaker, ½ cup (48 g)	210	8	34	3.5	15	0

BREADS & CEREALS

FOOD/PORTION SIZE	CAL	FAT Total (g)	FAT As % of Cal	SAT FAT Total (g)	SAT FAT As % of Cal	CHOL (mg)
Product 19, Kellogg's, 1 cup, 1.1 oz (30 g)	110	0	0	0	0	0
Puffed Rice, Quaker, 1 cup (14 g)	50	0	0	0	0	0
Puffed Wheat, Quaker, 1¼ cups (15 g)	50	0	0	0	0	0
Raisin Bran, Kellogg's, 1 cup (61 g)	200	1.5	7	0	0	0
Raisin Bran, Post, 1 cup (59 g)	190	1	5	0	0	0
Rice Chex, Ralston Purina, 1 cup (31 g)	120	0	0	0	0	0
Rice Krispies, Kellogg's, 1¼ cups (33 g)	120	0	0	0	0	0
Shredded Wheat, Nabisco, 2 biscuits (46 g)	160	<1	<3	0	0	0
Shredded Wheat, Spoon Size, Nabisco, 1 cup (49 g)	170	<1	<3	0	0	0
Special K, Kellogg's, 1 cup, 1.1 oz (30 g)	110	0	0	0	0	0
Sugar Frosted Flakes, Kellogg's, ¾ cup, 1.1 oz (30 g)	120	0	0	0	0	0
Trix, General Mills, 1 cup (30 g)	120	<2	<11	0	0	0
Wheat Chex, Ralston Purina, ¾ cup (50 g)	190	1	5	0	0	0
Wheaties, General Mills, 1 cup (30 g)	110	1	8	0	0	0
CEREALS, HOT						
Corn Grits, Regular/Quick, Original, Quaker Instant Grits, 1 packet (28 g)	100	0	0	0	0	0
Cream of Wheat, Instant, Nabisco, 1 packet (28 g)	100	0	0	0	0	0
Oat Bran, Quaker Oats, ½ cup (40 g)	150	3	18	1	6	0

FOOD/PORTION SIZE	CAL	FAT Total (g)	FAT As % of Cal	SAT FAT Total (g)	SAT FAT As % of Cal	CHOL (mg)
Oats, Instant, Apple Cinnamon, Quaker Oats, 1 packet (35 g)	130	<2	<10	<1	<3	0
Oats, Instant, Bananas & Cream, Quaker Oats, 1 packet (35 g)	140	<3	<16	<1	<3	0
Oats, Instant, Blueberries & Cream, Quaker Oats, 1 packet (35 g)	130	<3	<17	<1	<3	0
Oats, Instant, Cinnamon Toast, Quaker Oats, 1 packet (35 g)	130	2	14	0	0	0
Oats, Instant, Maple & Brown Sugar, Quaker Oats, 1 packet (43 g)	160	2	11	<1	<3	0
Oats, Instant, Peaches & Cream, Quaker Oats, 1 packet (35 g)	130	2	14	<1	<3	0
Oats, Instant, Raisin Date Walnut, Quaker Oats, 1 packet (37 g)	130	<3	<17	<1	<3	0
Oats, Instant, Regular, Quaker Oats, dry, 1 packet (28 g)	100	2	18	0	0	0
Oats, Instant, Strawberries & Cream, Quaker Oats, 1 packet (35 g)	130	2	14	<1	<3	0
Oats, Old Fashioned, Quaker Oats, ½ cup cooked (40 g dry)	150	3	18	<1	<3	0
CRACKERS						
Cheese, Plain, 1-in. Square, Cheese Nips, Nabisco, 29 crackers (30 g)	150	6	36	1.5	9	0
Cheese, Sandwich, Peanut Butter, Keebler, 1 pkg (38 g)	190	9	43	2	9	<5
Graham, Honey, Honey Maid, Nabisco, 8 crackers (28 g)	120	3	23	.5	4	0

BREADS & CEREALS

FOOD/PORTION SIZE	CAL	FAT Total (g)	FAT As % of Cal	SAT FAT Total (g)	SAT FAT As % of Cal	CHOL (mg)
Graham, plain, 2½-in. square, 2 crackers	60	1	15	<1	<6	0
Ritz, Nabisco, 5 crackers (16 g)	80	4	45	<1	<6	0
Rye Wafers, Whole-Grain, Original Crispbread, Wasa, 1 slice (14 g)	45	0	0	0	0	0
Rykrisp, Natural, 2 crackers (15 g)	60	0	0	0	0	0
Saltines, 4 crackers	50	1	18	<1	<9	4
Saltines, Salerno, 5 crackers (15 g)	60	2	30	0	0	0
Town House, 50% Reduced Sodium, Keebler, 5 crackers (16 g)	80	<5	<51	1	11	0
Wheatables, 50% Reduced Fat, Savory Original, Keebler, 29 crackers (30 g)	130	<4	<24	1	7	0
Wheat Thins, Original, Nabisco, 16 crackers (29 g)	140	6	39	1	6	0
Whole Wheat Wafers, Triscuit, Nabisco, 7 wafers	140	5	32	1	6	0

MUFFINS

FOOD/PORTION SIZE	CAL	FAT Total (g)	FAT As % of Cal	SAT FAT Total (g)	SAT FAT As % of Cal	CHOL (mg)
Apple Cinnamon, Otis Spunkmeyer, ½ muffin (57 g)	220	11	45	2	8	35
Blueberry, Frozen, Wholesome Choice, Pepperidge Farm, 1 muffin (54 g)	140	2.5	16	0	0	0
Blueberry, Mix, Jiffy, ¼ cup mix	160	5	28	2	11	0
Blueberry, Muffin Mix, Duncan Hines, ¼ cup mix	150	4.5	27	1	6	0
Blueberry, Wild, Betty Crocker, regular recipe, 1 muffin (40 g mix)	140	<2	<10	<1	<3	0
Bran, mix, 1 muffin	140	4	26	1	6	28

FOOD/PORTION SIZE	CAL	FAT		SAT FAT		CHOL (mg)
		Total (g)	As % of Cal	Total (g)	As % of Cal	
Bran, Mix, Krusteaz, ⅓ cup mix	190	5	24	1	5	0
Chocolate Chocolate Chip, 97% Fat Free, Frozen, Weight Watchers, 1 muffin (71 g)	190	2	9	1	5	0
English, Honey Wheat, Thomas', 1 muffin (57 g)	110	1	8	0	0	0
English, Original, Wonder, 1 muffin (57 g)	120	1	8	0	0	0
English, plain, enriched, 1 muffin	140	1	6	<1	<2	0
English, Thomas', 1 muffin (57 g)	120	1	8	0	0	0

ROLLS

FOOD/PORTION SIZE	CAL	FAT		SAT FAT		CHOL (mg)
Dinner Rolls, Crescent, Pillsbury, 2 rolls (57 g)	200	11	50	<3	<11	0
Dinner Rolls, Enriched, Country Style, Pepperidge Farm, 3 rolls (57 g)	150	3	18	1	6	0
Frankfurter, Brownberry, 1 roll (43 g)	110	2	16	0	0	0
Frankfurter/hamburger, enriched commercial, 1 roll	115	2	16	<1	<4	tr
Hamburger, Enriched, Butternut, 1 bun (49 g)	140	2	13	.5	3	0
Hard, enriched, commercial, 1 roll	155	2	12	<1	<2	tr
Hard, Jumbo Rolls, S. Rosen, 1 roll (60 g)	160	4	23	0	0	0
Hoagie/submarine, enriched commercial, 1 roll	400	8	18	2	5	tr
Kaiser, Francisco International, Brownberry, 1 roll (57 g)	170	1	5	0	0	0

BREADS & CEREALS

FOOD/PORTION SIZE	CAL	FAT		SAT FAT		CHOL (mg)
		Total (g)	As % of Cal	Total (g)	As % of Cal	
MISCELLANEOUS						
Bagel, Cinnamon Raisin, Thomas', 1 bagel (104 g)	280	2	6	1	3	0
Bagel, Egg, Lender's, 1 bagel (81 g)	220	2.5	10	.5	2	15
Bagel, Plain, Lender's, 1 bagel (81 g)	210	1.5	6	0	0	0
Bagel, Plain, Thomas', 1 bagel (61 g)	150	1	6	0	0	0
Bran, Unprocessed, Hodgson Mill, ¼ cup dry (15 g)	30	0	0	0	0	0
Breadsticks, Refrigerated, Pillsbury, 1 stick (39 g)	110	<3	<20	<1	<4	0
Crescent, Butter, European Bake Shoppe, Pepperidge Farm, 1 roll (30 g)	110	5	41	3	25	15
Croissant, with enriched flour, 1 croissant	235	12	46	4	15	13
Melba toast, plain, 1 piece	20	tr	na	<1	<5	0
Melba Toast, White, Old London, 5 pieces (15 g)	50	0	0	0	0	0
Pancakes & Waffle Mix, Original, Aunt Jemima, ⅓ cup mix	160	.5	3	0	0	0
Stuffing, Country Garden Herb, Pepperidge Farm, ½ cup (34 g)	150	5	30	1	6	0
Stuffing Mix, Chicken Flavored, Stove Top One Step, about ½ cup mix (28 g)	120	3	23	<1	<4	0
Stuffing Mix, Croutettes, Kellogg's, approx. 1 cup (35 g)	120	0	0	0	0	0
Taco Shell, Lawry's, 2 shells (23 g)	120	6	45	1.5	11	0
Tortilla, Corn, Refrigerated, Azteca, 2 tortillas (34 g)	90	1	10	0	0	0

FOOD/PORTION SIZE	CAL	FAT Total (g)	FAT As % of Cal	SAT FAT Total (g)	SAT FAT As % of Cal	CHOL (mg)
Tortillas, Flour, 7-inch, Azteca, 2 tortillas (48 g)	160	3	17	.5	3	0
Waffles, Kellogg's Special K, Eggo, 2 waffles (58 g)	140	0	0	0	0	0
Wheat Bran, Toasted, Kretschmer, ¼ cup (16 g)	30	1	30	0	0	0

Candy

FOOD/PORTION SIZE	CAL	FAT Total (g)	FAT As % of Cal	SAT FAT Total (g)	SAT FAT As % of Cal	CHOL (mg)
Baby Ruth, 1 bar (2.1 oz)	280	12	39	7	23	0
Butterfinger Bar, Kingsize, ⅓ bar (36 g)	170	7	37	4	19	0
Caramels, Kraft, 5 pieces, (41 g)	170	3.5	19	1	5	<5
Chocolate, Sweet Dark, Hershey's, 3 blocks (37 g)	200	12	54	7	32	0
Crunch, Nestlé, 1 bar (44 g)	230	12	47	7	27	5
Dessert Mints, Brach's, 37 pieces (40 g)	160	0	0	0	0	0
Fudge, chocolate, plain, 1 oz	117	3	23	2	15	1
Gum Drops, Spice Drops, Brach's, 12 pieces (39 g)	130	0	0	0	0	0
Hard Candy, Jolly Rancher, 3 pieces (18 g)	70	0	0	0	0	0
Jelly Beans, Brach's, 14 pieces (39 g)	140	0	0	0	0	0
Jet-Puffed Marshmallows, Kraft, 5 marshmallows (34 g)	110	0	0	0	0	0
Kisses, Hershey's, 8 pieces (39 g)	210	12	51	8	34	10
Kit-Kat, 1 bar	220	12	49	8	33	5
M & M's Peanut Chocolate Candies, ¼ cup, 1.5 oz	220	11	45	4.5	18	5

CANDY

FOOD/PORTION SIZE	CAL	FAT Total (g)	FAT As % of Cal	SAT FAT Total (g)	SAT FAT As % of Cal	CHOL (mg)
M & M's Plain Chocolate Candies, ¼ cup, 1.5 oz	210	9	39	6	26	5
Marshmallows, Miniature, Kraft, ½ cup (25 g)	80	0	0	0	0	0
Milk Chocolate, Plain, Hershey's, 3 blocks (42 g)	200	12	54	7	32	10
Milk Chocolate, with Almonds, Hershey's, 3 blocks (37 g)	210	13	56	6	26	5
Milk Chocolate, with Peanuts, Double Dippers, Brach's, 15 pieces (40 g)	220	14	57	6	25	5
Milky Way Bar, 1 bar (61 g)	280	11	35	5	16	5
Peanut Brittle, Sophie Mae, about ¼ cup, 1.4 oz	180	5	25	1	5	0
Peanut Butter Cups, Reese's, 2 pieces (34 g)	190	11	52	4	19	<5
Snickers, Fun Size, 2 bars (40 g)	190	10	47	3.5	17	5
Snickers, Miniature, 4 pieces (36 g)	170	9	48	3.5	19	5

Cheese

FOOD/PORTION SIZE	CAL	FAT Total (g)	FAT As % of Cal	SAT FAT Total (g)	SAT FAT As % of Cal	CHOL (mg)
American, Sharp, Processed Slices, Old English, Kraft, 1 slice (28 g)	110	9	74	5	49	30
American, Singles, Processed Cheese Food, Borden, 1 slice (21 g)	70	5	64	3	39	20
American, Singles, Processed Cheese Food, Deluxe, Kraft, 1 slice (21 g)	80	7	79	4.5	51	20

CHEESE

FOOD/PORTION SIZE	CAL	FAT Total (g)	FAT As % of Cal	SAT FAT Total (g)	SAT FAT As % of Cal	CHOL (mg)
American, Singles, Processed Cheese Food, Fat Free, Healthy Choice, 1 slice (21 g)	30	0	0	0	0	<5
American, Singles, Processed Cheese Food, Kraft, 1 slice (21 g)	70	5	64	3.5	45	15
American, Singles, Processed Cheese Food, Reduced Fat, 2% Milk, Kraft, 1 slice (21 g)	50	3	54	2	36	10
American, Singles, Processed Cheese Food, The Big!, Borden, 1 slice (24 g)	80	6	68	4	45	20
Blue, Crumbled, Treasure Cave, 1 oz (30 g)	110	9	74	6	49	25
Blue, Treasure Cave, 1 oz (30 g)	110	9	74	6	49	25
Camembert, Tradition de Belmont, 1 oz (28 g)	90	8	80	3	30	15
Cheddar, Extra Sharp, Cold Pack Cheese Food, Cracker Barrel, Kraft, 1 oz (28 g)	110	9	74	6	49	30
Cheddar, Mild, Reduced Fat, Kraft, ⅛ pack, 1 oz (28 g)	90	6	60	4	40	20
Cheddar, Mild, Shredded, Sargento, ¼ cup (28 g)	110	9	74	6	49	30
Cheddar, Natural, Kraft, 1 oz (28 g)	110	9	74	6	49	30
Cheddar, Port Wine, Cheese Log with Almonds, Kaukauna, 2 tbsp (28 g)	100	7	63	3.5	32	20
Cheddar, Port Wine, Cold Pack Cheese Food, Kaukauna, 2 tbsp (28 g)	90	7	70	3	30	20
Cheddar, Sharp, Cheese Ball with Almonds, Kaukauna, 2 tbsp (28 g)	100	7	63	3.5	32	20

CHEESE

FOOD/PORTION SIZE	CAL	FAT Total (g)	FAT As % of Cal	SAT FAT Total (g)	SAT FAT As % of Cal	CHOL (mg)
Cheddar, Sharp, Cold Pack Cheese Food, Kaukauna, 2 tbsp (28 g)	90	7	70	3	30	20
Cheddar, Sharp, Processed Cheese Product, Singles, Kraft Free, 1 slice (21 g)	35	0	0	0	0	0
Cheddar, Sharp, Reduced Fat, Kraft, 1 oz (28 g)	90	6	60	4	40	20
Cheese Spread, Processed, Mild Mexican, Velveeta, Kraft, 1 oz (28 g)	90	6	60	4.5	45	20
Cheese Spread, Processed, Velveeta, 1 oz (28 g)	80	6	68	4	45	20
Cottage, Fat Free, Light n' Lively Free, ½ cup (124 g)	80	0	0	0	0	5
Cottage, Fat Free, Small Curd, Breakstone's, ½ cup (124 g)	80	0	0	0	0	5
Cottage, Lowfat, Light n' Lively, ½ cup (115 g)	80	1	11	1	11	10
Cottage, Lowfat, Small Curd, Breakstone's, ½ cup (119 g)	90	2.5	25	1.5	15	15
Cream Cheese, Fat Free, Philadelphia Brand, 1 oz (28 g)	25	0	0	0	0	<5
Cream Cheese, Garden Vegetable, Fat Free, Soft, Philadelphia Brand Free, 2 tbsp (33 g)	35	0	0	0	0	<5
Cream Cheese, Philadelphia Brand, 1 oz (28 g)	100	10	90	6	54	30
Cream Cheese, Plain, Whipped, Philadelphia Brand, 3 tbsp (28 g)	100	11	99	7	63	35
Cream Cheese, Soft, Philadelphia Brand Free, 2 tbsp (33 g)	35	0	0	0	0	<5

FOOD/PORTION SIZE	CAL	FAT Total (g)	FAT As % of Cal	SAT FAT Total (g)	SAT FAT As % of Cal	CHOL (mg)
Cream Cheese Soft, Light, Philadelphia Brand, 2 tbsp (32 g)	70	5	64	3.5	45	15
Cream Cheese, Strawberry, Fat Free, Soft, Philadelphia Brand Free, 2 tbsp (33 g)	45	0	0	0	0	<5
Cream Cheese, Strawberry, Soft, Philadelphia Brand, 2 tbsp (32 g)	100	9	81	6	54	30
Cream Cheese, with Chives, Whipped, Philadelphia Brand, 3 tbsp (31 g)	100	9	81	6	54	30
Cream Cheese, with Chives & Onion, Soft, Philadelphia Brand, 2 tbsp (31 g)	110	10	82	7	57	30
Cream Cheese, with Pineapple, Soft, Philadelphia Brand, 2 tbsp (32 g)	100	9	81	6	54	30
Cream Cheese, with Salmon, Soft, Philadelphia Brand, 2 tbsp (31 g)	100	9	81	6	54	30
Feta, Crumbled, Treasure Cave, 1 oz (30 g)	80	6	68	4	45	20
Monterey Jack, Natural, Kraft, 1 oz (28 g)	110	9	74	6	49	30
Mozzarella, Part-Skim Milk, Kraft, 1 oz (28 g)	80	5	56	3.5	39	20
Mozzarella, Shredded, Part-Skim Milk, Kraft, ¼ cup (30 g)	90	6	60	4	40	20
Mozzarella, Shredded, Reduced Fat, Light, Sargento, ¼ cup (28 g)	70	3.5	45	2.5	32	10
Mozzarella, Truly Lite, Frigo, 1 oz (28 g)	60	<3	<38	<2	<23	15
Mozzarella, Whole Milk, Sorrento, 1 oz (30 g)	90	7	70	4.5	45	25

CHEESE

FOOD/PORTION SIZE	CAL	FAT Total (g)	FAT As % of Cal	SAT FAT Total (g)	SAT FAT As % of Cal	CHOL (mg)
Muenster, 1 oz	104	8	69	4	35	27
Parmesan, Grated, Kraft, 2 tbsp (5 g)	20	1.5	68	1	45	5
Provolone, Auricchio Americano, 1 oz (28.3 g)	103	na	na	na	na	na
Ricotta, Fat Free, Frigo, ¼ cup (62 g)	45	0	0	0	0	5
Ricotta, Part-Skim Milk, Frigo, ¼ cup (62 g)	100	7	63	5	45	35
Ricotta, Whole Milk, Sorrento, ¼ cup (62 g)	110	8.5	70	6.5	53	35
Romano, Grated, Kraft, 2 tbsp (5 g)	25	1.5	54	1	36	5
Swiss, Block, County Line, 1 oz (30 g)	110	8	65	5	41	30
Swiss, Natural, Kraft, 1 slice (23 g)	90	6	60	4	40	20
Swiss, Singles, Processed Cheese Food, Kraft, 1 slice (21 g)	70	5	64	3	39	15
Swiss, Singles, Processed, Cheese Product, Nonfat, Kraft Free, 1 slice (21 g)	30	0	0	0	0	<5
Swiss Flavor, Processed, Fat Free, Borden, 1 slice (21 g)	30	0	0	0	0	0

Cream & Creamers

FOOD/PORTION SIZE	CAL	FAT Total (g)	FAT As % of Cal	SAT FAT Total (g)	SAT FAT As % of Cal	CHOL (mg)
Cool Whip, Extra Creamy, Dairy Recipe, Whipped Topping, Birds Eye, 2 tbsp (9 g)	30	2	60	2	60	0

FOOD/PORTION SIZE	CAL.	FAT Total (g)	FAT As % of Cal.	SAT. FAT Total (g)	SAT. FAT As % of Cal.	CHOL. (mg)
Cool Whip, Lite, Whipped Topping, Birds Eye, 2 tbsp (8 g)	20	1	45	1	45	0
Cool Whip, Non-Dairy, Whipped Topping, Birds Eye, 2 tbsp (8 g)	25	<2	<54	<2	<54	0
Cream, Instant, Real Whipped, Heavy Cream, Sweetened, Deluxe, Reddi Whip (pressurized), 2 tbsp (8 g)	30	3	90	2	60	10
Cream, sweet, half-and-half, 1 tbsp	20	2	90	2	90	6
Cream, sweet, light/ coffee/table, 1 tbsp	30	3	90	2	60	10
Cream, sweet, whipping, unwhipped, heavy, 1 tbsp	50	6	100	4	72	21
Cream, sweet, whipping, unwhipped, light, 1 tbsp	44	5	100	3	61	17
Cream, whipped topping, pressurized, 1 tbsp	10	1	90	<1	<72	0
Creamer, Nondairy, Coffee-mate, 1 tbsp (15 ml)	20	1	45	0	0	0
Creamer, sweet, imitation, liquid, 1 tbsp	20	1	45	<2	<63	0
Sour Cream, Fat Free, Breakstone's Free, 2 tbsp (32 g)	35	0	0	0	0	<5
Sour Cream, Land O Lakes, 1 tbsp	20	1	45	1	45	1
Sour Cream, Light, Land O Lakes, 2 tbsp (31 g)	35	2	51	1.5	39	10
Whipped Cream, Light, Dairy Whip, Kraft (pressurized), 2 tbsp (5 g)	10	1	90	1	90	<5
Whipped Topping Mix, Dream Whip (prepared with 2% milk & vanilla), 1/16 pouch (2.5 g)	20	na	na	na	na	na

Eggs

FOOD/PORTION SIZE	CAL	FAT Total (g)	FAT As % of Cal	SAT FAT Total (g)	SAT FAT As % of Cal	CHOL (mg)
Egg Beaters, Fleischmann's, ¼ cup (61 g)	30	0	0	0	0	0
Egg Substitute, Second Nature, ¼ cup (60 ml)	40	0	0	0	0	0
Large, fried in butter, 1 egg	83	7	76	3	33	278
Large, hard-cooked, 1 egg	80	6	68	2	23	213
Large, poached, 1 egg	80	6	68	2	23	213
Large, raw, white only, 1 white	15	0	0	0	0	0
Large, raw, whole, 1 egg	80	6	68	2	23	213
Large, raw, yolk only, 1 yolk	65	6	83	2	28	213
Scrambled, with milk, cooked in margarine, 1 egg	100	7	63	2	18	215

Fast Foods

FOOD/PORTION SIZE	CAL	FAT Total (g)	FAT As % of Cal	SAT FAT Total (g)	SAT FAT As % of Cal	CHOL (mg)
ARBY'S						
Beef N' Cheddar Sandwich, 1 order	510	27	48	8	14	50
Chicken Breast Fillet Sandwich, 1 order	450	23	46	3	6	45
Dressing, Buttermilk, 1 packet	350	39	100	6	15	5
Dressing, Honey French, 1 packet	320	27	76	4	11	0
French Dip Sub, 1 order	470	21	40	8	15	60
French Fries, 1 order	250	13	47	3	11	0
Italian Sub, 1 order	660	36	49	13	18	80
Light Roast Beef Deluxe Sandwich, 1 order	290	10	31	3.5	11	40
Light Roast Chicken Deluxe Sandwich, 1 order	280	7	23	2	6	33

FOOD/PORTION SIZE	CAL	FAT Total (g)	FAT As % of Cal	SAT FAT Total (g)	SAT FAT As % of Cal	CHOL (mg)
Light Roast Turkey Deluxe Sandwich, 1 order	260	6	21	1.5	5	35
Roast Beef Sandwich, Regular, 1 order	380	18	43	7	17	45
Salad, Garden, 1 order	120	5	38	3	23	15
Salad, Roast Chicken, 1 order	200	7	32	3.5	16	45
Salad, Side, 1 order	25	0	0	0	0	0
Turkey Sub, 1 order	530	26	44	7	12	55

BURGER KING

Bacon Double Cheeseburger, 1 order	640	39	55	18	25	145
BK Big Fish Fillet Sandwich, 1 order	720	43	54	8	10	60
Broiled Chicken Salad, 1 order	200	10	45	5	23	60
Cheeseburger, 1 order	380	19	45	9	21	55
Chicken BK Broiler Sandwich, 1 order	540	29	48	6	10	80
Croissan'wich with Bacon, 1 order	350	24	62	8	21	225
Croissan'wich with Ham, 1 order	350	22	57	7	18	230
Croissan'wich with Sausage, 1 order	530	41	70	14	24	255
French Fries, salted, medium, 1 order	400	20	45	5	11	0
French Toast Sticks, 1 order	500	27	49	7	13	0
Hamburger, 1 order	330	15	41	6	16	55
Onion Rings, 1 order	310	14	41	2	6	0
Pie, Apple, 1 order	310	15	44	3	9	0
Salad, Chef, 1 order	210	11	47	4	17	180
Whopper, 1 order	640	39	55	11	15	90
Whopper with Cheese, 1 order	730	46	57	16	20	115

FAST FOODS

FOOD/PORTION SIZE	CAL	FAT Total (g)	FAT As % of Cal	SAT FAT Total (g)	SAT FAT As % of Cal	CHOL (mg)
DAIRY QUEEN						
Banana Split, 1 order	510	11	19	8	14	30
Cone, Regular, Chocolate, 1 order	350	11	28	8	21	30
Fish Fillet Sandwich, 1 order	370	16	39	3	7	45
Fish Fillet Sandwich with Cheese, 1 order	420	21	45	6	13	60
Grilled Chicken Fillet Sandwich, 1 order	310	10	29	2.5	7	50
Hamburger, Single, 1 order	290	12	37	5	16	45
Heath Blizzard, Small, 1 order	560	23	37	11	18	40
Hot Dog, 1 order	240	14	53	5	19	25
Malt, Regular Vanilla, 1 order	610	14	21	8	12	45
Parfait, Peanut Buster, 1 order	710	32	41	10	13	30
Shake, Regular Chocolate, 1 order	540	14	23	8	13	45
Sundae, Regular Chocolate, 1 order	300	7	21	5	15	20
DOMINO'S						
Pizza, Cheese, Deep Dish, 12 inches, ¼ pizza	560	24	39	9	14	32
Pizza, Cheese, Thin Crust, 12 inches, ⅓ pizza	360	16	40	6	15	25
Pizza, Extra Cheese & Pepperoni, Deep Dish, 12 inches, ¼ pizza	670	33	44	13	17	55
Pizza, Ham, Hand-Tossed, 12 inches, ¼ pizza	360	10	25	4.5	11	25
Pizza, Ham, Thin Crust, 12 inches, ⅓ pizza	390	17	39	7	16	35
Pizza, Italian Sausage & Mushroom, Thin Crust, 12 inches, ⅓ pizza	440	21	43	9	18	40

FOOD/PORTION SIZE	CAL	FAT Total (g)	FAT As % of Cal	SAT FAT Total (g)	SAT FAT As % of Cal	CHOL (mg)
Pizza, Veggie, Deep Dish, 12 inches, ¼ pizza	580	25	39	9	14	35
KENTUCKY FRIED CHICKEN						
Biscuit, 1 order, 2 oz	200	12	54	3	14	2
Coleslaw, 1 order	110	6	49	1	8	<5
Extra Tasty Crispy, breast, 1 piece, 5.9 oz	470	28	54	7	13	80
Extra Tasty Crispy, drumstick, 1 piece, 2.4 oz	190	11	52	3	14	60
Extra Tasty Crispy, wing, 1 piece, 1.9 oz	200	13	59	4	18	45
Hot & Spicy, breast, 1 piece, 6.5 oz	530	35	59	8	14	110
Hot & Spicy, drumstick, 1 piece, 2.3 oz	190	11	52	3	14	50
Hot Wings, six wings, 4.8 oz	470	33	63	8	15	150
Kentucky Nuggets, six nuggets, 3.4 oz	280	18	58	4	13	65
Mashed Potatoes with Gravy, 1 order, 4.2 oz	110	5	41	.5	4	0
Quarter, breast & wing, Rotisserie Gold, 1 order, 6.2 oz	340	19	50	5	13	160
Quarter, breast & wing, Rotisserie Gold, w/o skin, 1 order, 4.1 oz	200	6	27	2	9	100
LONG JOHN SILVER'S						
Baked Chicken, Light Herb, 3.5 oz	120	4	30	1.5	11	60
Baked Fish, Lemon Crumb, 15.9 oz	150	1	6	<1	<4	110
Baked Fish (3 pieces), Lemon Crumb, with rice, beans, slaw and roll, 1 order	610	13	19	<2.5	<4	125

FAST FOODS

| FOOD/PORTION SIZE | CAL | FAT | | SAT FAT | | CHOL (mg) |
		Total (g)	As % of Cal	Total (g)	As % of Cal	
Chicken Plank, 2 pieces	240	12	45	3.5	13	30
Clams, 2 hushpuppies, fries and slaw, 1 order, 12.7 oz	990	52	47	11	10	75
Seafood Gumbo, with cod, 1 order, 7 oz	120	8	60	<3	<16	25

McDONALD'S

Big Mac, 1 order	510	26	46	9	16	75
Biscuit with Bacon, Egg, and Cheese, 1 order	450	27	54	9	18	240
Biscuit with Sausage, 1 order	430	29	61	9	19	35
Biscuit with Sausage and Egg, 1 order	520	35	61	10	17	245
Cheeseburger, 1 order	320	13	37	6	17	40
Chicken McNuggets, 6 pieces	300	18	54	3.5	11	65
Cone, Lowfat Frozen Yogurt, Vanilla, 1 cone	120	.5	3	0	0	5
Cookies, Chocolate Chip, 1 order	280	14	45	4	13	5
Cookies, McDonaldland, 1 order	260	9	31	2	7	0
Danish, Apple, 1 order	360	16	40	5	13	40
Danish, Cinnamon Raisin, 1 order	430	22	46	7	15	50
Danish, Raspberry, 1 order	400	16	36	5	11	45
Dressing, Lite Vinaigrette, 1 packet	50	2	36	0	0	0
Dressing, Ranch, 1 packet,	230	21	82	3	12	20
Egg McMuffin, 1 order	290	13	40	4.5	14	235
Eggs, Scrambled, 2 eggs	170	12	64	3.5	19	425
Filet-O-Fish Sandwich, 1 order	360	16	40	3.5	8	35
French Fries, small, 1 order	210	10	43	1.5	6	0
Hamburger, 1 order	270	9	30	3	10	30

FOOD/PORTION SIZE	CAL	FAT Total (g)	FAT As % of Cal	SAT FAT Total (g)	SAT FAT As % of Cal	CHOL (mg)
Hashbrowns, 1 order	130	8	55	1.5	10	0
Hotcakes with 2 pats margarine and syrup, 1 order	560	14	23	2.5	4	10
McLean Deluxe, 1 order	340	12	32	4.5	12	60
Pie, Apple, 1 order	290	15	47	35	11	0
Quarter Pounder, 1 order	420	20	43	8	17	70
Quarter Pounder with Cheese, 1 order	520	29	50	13	23	95
Salad, Chef, 1 order	210	11	47	4	17	180
Salad, Chicken, Chunky, 1 order	160	5	28	1.5	8	75
Salad, Garden, 1 order	80	4	45	1	11	140
Sauce, Barbecue, 1 packet	50	0	0	0	0	0
Sauce, Hot Mustard, 1 packet	60	3.5	53	0	0	5
Sauce, Sweet-n-Sour, 1 packet	50	0	0	0	0	0
Sausage McMuffin, 1 order	360	23	58	8	20	45
Sausage McMuffin with Egg, 1 order	440	29	59	10	20	255
Sausage Patty, 1 order	170	16	85	5	26	35
Shake, Chocolate, small, 1 order	350	6	15	3.5	9	25
Shake, Strawberry, small, 1 order	340	5	13	3.5	9	25
Shake, Vanilla, small, 1 order	310	5	15	3.5	10	25
Sundae, Vanilla, Lowfat Frozen Yogurt, 1 order	170	1	5	1	5	<5
Sundae Topping, Caramel, 1 order	140	2	13	1	6	0
Sundae Topping, Hot Fudge, 1 order	130	4	28	4	28	0
Sundae Topping, Strawberry, 1 order	80	0	0	0	0	0

FAST FOODS

FOOD/PORTION SIZE	CAL	FAT Total (g)	FAT As % of Cal	SAT FAT Total (g)	SAT FAT As % of Cal	CHOL (mg)
PIZZA HUT						
Pizza, Bigfoot Cheese, 1 slice	190	6	28	3	14	15
Pizza, Hand-Tossed, Cheese, 1 slice	240	7	26	4	15	25
Pizza, Hand-Tossed, Supreme, 1 slice	280	12	39	5	16	30
Pizza, Pan, Super Supreme, 1 slice	300	13	39	5	15	35
Pizza, Personal Pan, Pepperoni, 5-inch, 1 order	640	28	39	10	14	55
Pizza, Personal Pan, Supreme, 5-inch, 1 order	720	34	43	12	15	65
Pizza, Thin 'N Crispy, Pepperoni, 15-inch, 1 slice	220	10	41	4	16	25
Pizza, Thin 'N Crispy, Supreme, 15-inch, 1 slice	260	13	45	5	17	30
SUBWAY						
BMT Salad, 1 order	630	52	74	19	27	135
BMT Sub, Italian Roll, 12-inch, 1 order	980	55	51	20	18	135
Club Salad, 1 order	350	19	49	6	15	85
Club Sub, Italian Roll, 12-inch, 1 order	690	22	29	7	9	85
Cold Cut Combo Salad, 1 order	510	37	65	11	19	170
Cold Cut Combo Sub, Italian Roll, 12-inch, 1 order	850	40	42	12	13	170
Ham & Cheese Salad, 1 order	300	18	54	6	18	75
Ham & Cheese Sub, Italian Roll, 12-inch, 1 order	640	18	25	7	10	75
Meatball Sub, Italian Roll, 12-inch, 1 order	920	44	43	17	17	90
Roast Beef Salad, 1 order	340	20	53	7	19	75

FOOD/PORTION SIZE	CAL	FAT		SAT FAT		CHOL (mg)
		Total (g)	As % of Cal	Total (g)	As % of Cal	
Roast Beef Sub, Italian Roll, 12-inch, 1 order	690	23	30	8	10	75
Seafood & Crab Salad, 1 order	640	53	75	10	14	55
Seafood & Crab Sub, Italian Roll, 12-inch, 1 order	990	57	52	11	10	55
Steak & Cheese Sub, Honey Wheat Roll, 12-inch, 1 order	710	33	42	12	15	80
Tuna Salad, 1 order	760	68	81	12	14	85
Tuna Sub, Italian Roll, 12-inch, 1 order	1100	72	59	13	11	85
Turkey Breast Salad, 1 order	300	16	48	4.5	14	70
Turkey Breast Sub, Italian Roll, 12-inch, 1 order	640	19	27	6	8	70
Veggies & Cheese Sub, Italian Roll, 12-inch, 1 order	540	17	28	5	8	20
WENDY'S						
Chicken Club Sandwich, 1 order	520	25	43	6	10	75
Chicken Nuggets, 6 pieces	280	20	64	5	16	50
Chicken Sandwich, Grilled, 1 order	290	7	22	<2	<5	55
Chili, small, 1 order, 8 oz	190	6	28	<3	<9	40
Cookies, Chocolate Chip, 1 order	270	11	37	8	27	0
Fries, small, 1 order, 3.2 oz	240	12	45	<3	<9	0
Frosty Dairy Dessert, small, 1 order, 12 oz	340	10	26	5	13	0
Hamburger, Jr., 1 order	270	9	30	3	10	35
Hamburger, Kid's Meal, with White Bun, 1 order	270	9	30	3	10	35
Hamburger, Single, Plain, ¼ lb, 1 order	350	15	39	6	15	70
Nuggets Sauce, Barbeque, 1 packet	50	0	0	0	0	0

FAST FOODS

FOOD/PORTION SIZE	CAL	FAT Total (g)	FAT As % of Cal	SAT FAT Total (g)	SAT FAT As % of Cal	CHOL (mg)
Nuggets Sauce, Honey, 1 packet	45	0	0	0	0	0
Nuggets Sauce, Sweet & Sour, 1 packet	45	0	0	0	0	0
Nuggets Sauce, Sweet Mustard, 1 packet	50	1	18	0	0	0
Potato, Hot Stuffed Baked, Bacon & Cheese, 1 order	530	18	31	4	7	20
Potato, Hot Stuffed Baked, Broccoli & Cheese, 1 order	460	14	27	<3	<5	0
Potato, Hot Stuffed Baked, Cheese, 1 order	560	23	37	8	13	30
Potato, Hot Stuffed Baked, Chili & Cheese, 1 order	610	24	35	9	13	45
Potato, Hot Stuffed Baked, Plain, 1 order	310	0	0	0	0	0
Potato, Hot Stuffed Baked, Sour Cream & Chives, 1 order	380	6	15	4	10	15
Salad, Caesar (w/o dressing), 1 order	110	5	41	2	16	15
Salad, Deluxe Garden (w/o dressing), 1 order	110	6	50	1	8	0
Salad, Taco, 1 order	580	30	47	11	17	75

Fats & Oils

FOOD/PORTION SIZE	CAL	FAT Total (g)	FAT As % of Cal	SAT FAT Total (g)	SAT FAT As % of Cal	CHOL (mg)
Butter, Salted, Land O Lakes, 1 tbsp (14 g)	100	11	99	7	63	30
Butter, Unsalted, Land O Lakes, 1 tbsp (14 g)	100	11	99	8	72	30
Butter, Whipped, Land O Lakes, 1 tbsp (9 g)	60	7	100	5	75	20

CONSUMER GUIDE®

FOOD/PORTION SIZE	CAL	FAT Total (g)	FAT As % of Cal	SAT FAT Total (g)	SAT FAT As % of Cal	CHOL (mg)
Butter Buds, Butter Flavored Mix, 1 tbsp (14 g)	5	0	0	0	0	0
Buttery Spray, Weight Watchers, 1 spray (.28 g)	0	0	0	0	0	0
Cooking Spray, No-Stick, Aerosol, Wesson, 1 spray	0	0	0	0	0	0
Lard, 1 tbsp	115	13	100	5	39	12
Margarine, Soft, Diet, Parkay, 1 tbsp	50	6	100	1	18	0
Margarine, Soft, Parkay, 1 tbsp	100	11	99	2	18	0
Margarine, Spray, I Can't Believe It's Not Butter!, 1 spray	0	0	0	0	0	0
Margarine, Spreadable Stick, Shedd's Spread Country Crock, 1 tbsp	80	9	100	1.5	17	0
Margarine, Stick, Fleischmann's, 1 tbsp	100	11	99	2	18	0
Margarine, Stick, Land O Lakes, 1 tbsp	100	11	99	2	18	0
Margarine, Stick, Lower Fat, Fleischmann's, 1 tbsp	50	6	100	1	18	0
Margarine, Tub, Fat Free, Promise Ultra, 1 tbsp	5	0	0	0	0	0
Margarine, Tub, Land O Lakes, 1 tbsp	100	11	99	2	18	0
Margarine, Tub, Lower Fat, Fleischmann's, 1 tbsp	40	4.5	100	0	0	0
Margarine, Whipped, Parkay, 1 tbsp	70	7	90	1.5	19	0
Margarine Spread, Squeezable, I Can't Believe It's Not Butter!, 1 tbsp	90	10	100	2	20	0
Margarine Spread, Tub, Soft, Promise Ultra, 1 tbsp	35	4	100	0	0	0
Oil, Olive, Extra Virgin or Extra Light, Bertolli, 1 tbsp	130	14	97	2	14	na

FATS & OILS

FOOD/PORTION SIZE	CAL	FAT Total (g)	FAT As % of Cal	SAT FAT Total (g)	SAT FAT As % of Cal	CHOL (mg)
Oil, Olive, Wesson, 1 tbsp	120	14	100	1.5	11	0
Oil, peanut, 1 tbsp	125	14	100	2	14	0
Oil, soybean-cottonseed blend, hydrogenated, 1 tbsp	125	14	100	3	22	0
Oil, sunflower, 1 tbsp	125	14	100	1	7	0
Shortening, Wesson, 1 tbsp	110	12	98	3	25	0
Spread, Squeeze, Parkay, 1 tbsp	80	9	100	1.5	17	0
Spread, Stick, Move Over Butter, 1 tbsp	90	10	100	2	20	0
Spread, Stick, with Sweet Cream, Land O Lakes, 1 tbsp	90	10	100	2	20	0
Spread, Tub, Light, Land O Lakes Country Morning, 1 tbsp	50	6	100	2.5	45	5
Spread, Tub, Parkay, 1 tbsp	60	7	100	1.5	23	0
Spread, Tub, Whipped, Move Over Butter, 1 tbsp	60	7	100	1.5	23	0

Fish & Shellfish

FOOD/PORTION SIZE	CAL	FAT Total (g)	FAT As % of Cal	SAT FAT Total (g)	SAT FAT As % of Cal	CHOL (mg)
Catfish, breaded, fried, 3 oz	194	11	52	na	na	69
Catfish, skinless, baked w/o fat, 3 oz	120	5	38	1	8	60
Clams, Minced, Snow's, ¼ cup (55 g)	25	0	0	0	0	10
Clams, raw, meat only, 3 oz	65	1	14	<1	<4	43
Cod, Fillets, Frozen, Mrs. Paul's, 1 fillet (120 g) and 1 tsp relish mix (7 g)	250	11	40	3	11	40

FOOD/PORTION SIZE	CAL	FAT Total (g)	FAT As % of Cal	SAT FAT Total (g)	SAT FAT As % of Cal	CHOL (mg)
Cod, skinless, broiled w/o fat, 3 oz	90	1	10	0	0	50
Crabmeat, canned, 1 cup	135	3	20	<1	<3	135
Fillets, Crunchy, Country Style, Southern Fried, Gorton's, 2 fillets (104 g)	270	16	53	4	13	30
Fish Sticks, Battered, Frozen, Mrs. Paul's, 6 sticks	240	15	56	4	15	25
Flounder, baked, with lemon juice, w/o added fat, 3 oz	80	1	11	<1	<4	59
Haddock, breaded, fried, 3 oz	175	9	46	2	10	75
Haddock, skinless, baked w/o fat, 3 oz	90	1	10	0	0	60
Halibut, broiled, with butter, with lemon juice, 3 oz	140	6	39	3	19	62
Herring, pickled, 3 oz	190	13	62	4	19	85
Lobster, boiled, 3 oz	100	1	9	0	0	100
Mackerel, skinless, broiled w/o fat, 3 oz	190	12	57	3	14	60
Orange roughy, broiled, 3 oz	130	7	48	0	0	20
Oysters, breaded, fried, 1 oyster	90	5	50	1	10	35
Oysters, raw, meat only, 1 cup	160	4	23	1	6	120
Perch, ocean, breaded, fried, 1 fillet	185	11	54	3	15	66
Perch, Ocean, Fillets, Booth, 4 oz	100	2	18	0	0	45
Pollock, skinless, broiled w/o fat, 3 oz	100	1	9	0	0	80
Salmon, Pink, Chunk Style, in Spring Water, Chicken of the Sea, 2 oz (56 g)	60	2	30	1	15	20
Salmon, Pink, Chunk Style, in Water, Pillar Rock, 1/3 cup (56 g)	60	2	30	0	0	40
Salmon, red, baked, 3 oz	140	5	32	1	6	60

FISH & SHELLFISH

FOOD/PORTION SIZE	CAL	FAT Total (g)	FAT As % of Cal	SAT FAT Total (g)	SAT FAT As % of Cal	CHOL (mg)
Salmon, smoked, 3 oz	150	8	48	3	18	51
Sardines, canned in oil, drained, 3 oz	175	11	57	2	10	121
Sardines, Canned in Olive Oil, King Oscar, 1 can (85 g)	290	24	74	6	19	140
Sardines, Canned in Tomato Sauce, King Oscar, 1 can (85 g)	220	18	74	7	29	120
Scallops, breaded (frozen), reheated, 6 scallops	195	10	46	3	14	70
Scallops, broiled, 3 oz (5.7 large or 14 small)	150	1	6	0	0	60
Scallops, Fried, Frozen, Mrs. Paul's, 12 scallops	200	8	36	2	9	10
Shrimp, boiled, 3 oz	110	2	16	0	0	160
Shrimp, Canned, Medium, Chicken of the Sea, 2 oz	45	0	0	0	0	115
Shrimp, French fried, 7 medium, 3 oz	200	10	45	<3	<11	168
Snapper, cooked by dry heat, 3 oz	109	2	17	na	na	40
Sole, baked, with lemon juice, w/o added fat, 3 oz	90	1	10	tr	na	49
Surimi seafood, crab flavored, chunk style, ½ cup	84	tr	na	tr	na	25
Trout, Rainbow, skinless, broiled w/o fat, 3 oz	130	4	28	1	7	60
Tuna, Albacore, in Water, Bumble Bee, 2 oz (56 g)	100	5	45	2	18	30
Tuna, Chunk Light, in Spring Water, StarKist, ¼ cup (56 g, drained)	60	<1	<8	0	0	30
Tuna, Chunk Light, in Vegetable Oil, Bumble Bee, about ¼ cup (56 g)	110	6	49	1	8	30
Tuna, Chunk Light, in Water, Bumble Bee, 2 oz (56 g)	60	<1	<8	0	0	30
Whiting, Extra Fancy, Taste T Brand, 4 oz (112 g)	80	1.5	17	0	0	86

Frozen Desserts

FOOD/PORTION SIZE	CAL.	FAT Total (g)	FAT As % of Cal.	SAT. FAT Total (g)	SAT. FAT As % of Cal.	CHOL. (mg)
DAIRY						
Ice Cream, Butter Pecan, Breyers, ½ cup (70 g)	180	12	60	6	30	35
Ice Cream, Cherry Garcia, Ben & Jerry's, ½ cup	240	16	60	10	38	80
Ice Cream, Chocolate, Breyers, ½ cup (70 g)	160	8	45	6	34	30
Ice Cream, Chocolate Fudge, Nonfat, Edy's Grand, ½ cup	110	0	0	0	0	0
Ice Cream, French Vanilla, Light, Breyers, ½ cup	90	1.5	15	.5	5	30
Ice Cream, Strawberry, Natural, Breyers, ½ cup (70 g)	130	6	42	4	28	25
Ice Cream, Vanilla, Fat Free, Kemps, ½ cup	100	0	0	0	0	0
Ice Cream, Vanilla, Häagen-Dazs, ½ cup	270	18	60	11	37	120
Ice Cream, Vanilla, Natural, Breyers, ½ cup (70 g)	150	8	48	6	36	35
Ice Cream, Vanilla, Sealtest, ½ cup	140	7	45	5	32	30
Ice Cream, Vanilla/Chocolate/Strawberry, Sealtest, ½ cup	140	6	39	4	26	25
Ice milk, vanilla, hardened, 1 cup	185	6	29	4	19	18
Ice milk, vanilla, soft serve, 1 cup	225	5	20	3	12	13
Sherbet, Pink Lemonade, Edy's, ½ cup	130	1.5	10	1	7	4
Sorbet, Georgia Peach, Chunky, Real Fruit, ½ cup	110	1	8	.5	4	5
Sorbet, Peach, Whole Fruit, Edy's, ½ cup	130	0	0	0	0	0

FROZEN DESSERTS

FOOD/PORTION SIZE	CAL	FAT Total (g)	FAT As % of Cal	SAT FAT Total (g)	SAT FAT As % of Cal	CHOL (mg)
SPECIALTY BARS						
Chocolate with Dark Chocolate, Dove, 1 bar	260	17	59	10	35	25
Cone, Vanilla Fudge, Nestlé 1 cone	360	20	50	10	25	20
Cookies & Cream, Edy's Grand, 1 bar	260	17	59	9	31	25
Fruit Bars, all flavors, Edy's, 1 bar	90	0	0	0	0	0
Fruit Juice Bars, Light, Welch's, all flavors, 1 bar	25	0	0	0	0	0
Pudding Snacks, Chocolate, Jell-O, 1 snack (113 g)	160	5	28	2	11	0
Sandwich Bar, Vanilla, Häagen-Dazs, 1 bar	260	13	45	8	28	65
Toasted Almond, Good Humor, 1 bar	170	9	48	2.5	13	10
Vanilla & Milk Chocolate, Classics, Good Humor, 1 bar	200	13	59	9	41	15
Vanilla with Dark Chocolate, Dove, 1 bar	260	17	59	11	38	10
Vanilla with Dark Chocolate, Eskimo Pie, 1 pie	160	11	62	8	45	10

Frozen Entrées & Sandwiches

FOOD/PORTION SIZE	CAL	FAT Total (g)	FAT As % of Cal	SAT FAT Total (g)	SAT FAT As % of Cal	CHOL (mg)
MEAT ENTRÉES						
Lasagne with Meat & Sauce, Stouffer's, 1 pkg (297 g)	360	13	33	5	13	50

FOOD/PORTION SIZE	CAL	FAT		SAT FAT		CHOL (mg)
		Total (g)	As % of Cal	Total (g)	As % of Cal	
Oriental Beef, with Vegetables and Rice, Lean Cuisine, 1 meal (255 g)	210	4	17	1.5	6	30
Pork Rib, Boneless, Hungry Man, Swanson, 1 meal (400 g)	760	37	44	13	15	90
Pot Roast, Yankee, Hungry Man, Swanson, 1 meal (454 g)	400	11	25	3	7	45
Salisbury Steak Dinner, Classic, Healthy Choice, 1 meal	280	8	26	3	10	30
Salisbury Steak, Hungry Man, Swanson, 1 meal (461 g)	590	32	49	17	26	80
Salisbury Steak, Lean Cuisine, 1 meal (269 g)	270	8	27	3.5	12	60
Spaghetti, with Meat Sauce, Lean Cuisine, 1 meal (326 g)	300	4	12	1	3	15

MISCELLANEOUS

FOOD/PORTION SIZE	CAL	Total (g)	As % of Cal	Total (g)	As % of Cal	CHOL (mg)
Angel Hair Pasta, with Vegetables and Marinara Sauce, Lean Cuisine, 1 meal (283 g)	210	4	17	1	4	0
Bowtie Pasta and Mushrooms Marsala, Weight Watchers, 1 meal (273 g)	280	9	29	3.5	11	10
Cheddar Bake with Pasta & Vegetables, Lean Cuisine, 1 pkg (255 g)	250	6	22	2.5	9	10
Cheese Cannelloni, Lean Cuisine, 1 pkg (258 g)	240	5	19	3	11	22
Cheese Ravioli, Lean Cuisine, 1 pkg (240 g)	240	7	26	3	11	50
Chicken Chow Mein, with Rice, Lean Cuisine, 1 meal (255 g)	210	5	21	1	4	35

FROZEN ENTRÉES & SANDWICHES

FOOD/PORTION SIZE	CAL	FAT Total (g)	FAT As % of Cal	SAT FAT Total (g)	SAT FAT As % of Cal	CHOL (mg)
Chicken Noodle Dinner, On-Cor, 1 cup (151 g)	140	5	32	2	13	15
Fettucini Primavera, Lean Cuisine, 1 entrée (283 g)	260	8	28	2.5	9	15
Lasagne, Classic Cheese, Lean Cuisine, 1 pkg (255 g)	290	6	19	3	9	30
Macaroni & Cheese, Magical, Kid Cuisine, 1 meal	410	13	29	5	45	15
Macaroni & Cheese, Lean Cuisine, 1 meal (255 g)	270	7	23	3.5	12	20
Pasta Shells Marinara, Classic, Healthy Choice, 1 meal	370	4	10	2	5	25
Teriyaki Stir-Fry, with Pasta, Chicken and Vegetables, Lunch Express, Lean Cuisine, 1 meal (255 g)	260	5	17	1	3	30
PIZZAS						
Pizza, Cheese, Sausage and Mushroom, Original, Tombstone, ⅕ pizza (132 g)	310	15	44	7	20	30
Pizza, Cheese Party, Totino's, ½ pizza (139 g)	320	14	39	5	14	20
Pizza, Deluxe French Bread, Lean Cuisine, 1 pizza (173 g)	330	6	16	2.5	7	30
Pizza, Vegetable, Tombstone Light, ⅕ pizza (131 g)	240	7	26	<3	<9	10
Pizza, with Cheese, Pirate, Kid Cuisine, 1 meal	430	11	23	3	6	20
POULTRY ENTRÉES						
Bow Tie Pasta & Chicken, Lean Cuisine (269 g)	270	6	20	<2	<5	60

FOOD/PORTION SIZE	CAL.	FAT		SAT. FAT		CHOL. (mg)
		Total (g)	As % of Cal.	Total (g)	As % of Cal.	
Chicken & Rice, with Mesquite-Style Sauce, Lean 'n Tasty, Michelina's, 1 meal (227 g)	280	3	10	.5	2	20
Chicken Dijon Dinner, Healthy Choice, 1 meal	280	4	13	<2	<5	30
Chicken Fettucini, with Broccoli, Lunch Express Lean Cuisine, 1 meal (290 g)	290	8	25	3.5	11	40
Chicken Fiesta, with Rice and Vegetables, Lean Cuisine, 1 meal (240 g)	260	5	17	.5	2	30
Chicken Parmigiana Dinner, Healthy Choice, 1 meal	300	4	12	2	6	35
Chicken Pesto with Penne, Lean 'n Tasty, Michelina's, 1 meal (227 g)	290	6	19	3.5	11	35
Pot Pie, Chicken, Lean Cuisine, 1 meal (269 g)	320	10	28	2.5	7	35
Turkey, Hungry Man, Swanson, 1 meal (475 g)	530	17	29	6	10	45

SEAFOOD ENTRÉES

FOOD/PORTION SIZE	CAL.	Total (g)	As % of Cal.	Total (g)	As % of Cal.	CHOL. (mg)
Baked Fish with Cheddar Shells, Lean Cuisine, 1 meal (255 g)	260	8	28	2	7	50
Fish Fillet, Italian Herb, Gorton's, 1 fillet (108 g)	130	6	42	1	7	60
Fish Fillet, Lemon Pepper, Gorton's, 1 fillets (108 g)	120	6	45	1	8	60
Pasta & Tuna Casserole, Lean Cuisine, 1 entrée (272 g)	280	6	19	2	6	20

STUFFED SANDWICHES

FOOD/PORTION SIZE	CAL.	Total (g)	As % of Cal.	Total (g)	As % of Cal.	CHOL. (mg)
Barbecue, Hot Pockets Stuffed Sandwiches, 1 piece (128 g)	340	12	32	5	13	25

FROZEN ENTRÉES & SANDWICHES

FOOD/PORTION SIZE	CAL	FAT Total (g)	FAT As % of Cal	SAT FAT Total (g)	SAT FAT As % of Cal	CHOL (mg)
Beef & Cheddar, Hot Pockets Stuffed Sandwiches, 1 piece (128 g)	360	18	45	9	23	50
Chicken Fajita, Lean Pockets Stuffed Sandwiches, 1 piece (128 g)	260	8	28	3	10	40
Ham 'N Cheese, Hot Pockets Stuffed Sandwiches, 1 piece (128 g)	340	15	40	7	19	45
Pizza Deluxe, Lean Pockets Stuffed Sandwiches, 1 piece (128 g)	290	8	25	3	9	25
Turkey, Broccoli & Cheese, Lean Pockets Stuffed Sandwiches, 1 piece (128 g)	260	8	28	3	10	35
Turkey & Ham with Cheddar, Lean Pockets Stuffed Sandwiches, 1 piece (128 g)	270	8	27	3	10	35
Turkey & Ham with Cheese, Hot Pockets Stuffed Sandwiches, 1 piece (128 g)	320	13	37	6	17	35

Fruit

FOOD/PORTION SIZE	CAL	FAT Total (g)	FAT As % of Cal	SAT FAT Total (g)	SAT FAT As % of Cal	CHOL (mg)
Apples, dried, sulfured, 10 rings	155	tr	na	tr	na	0
Apples, raw, unpeeled, 3¼-in. diameter, 1 apple	125	1	7	<1	na	0

FOOD/PORTION SIZE	CAL	FAT Total (g)	FAT As % of Cal	SAT FAT Total (g)	SAT FAT As % of Cal	CHOL (mg)
Apple Sauce, Bottled, Chunky, with Brown Sugar & Cinnamon, Homestyle, Mott's, ½ cup (123 g)	100	0	0	0	0	0
Apple Sauce, Bottled, Cinnamon, Naturally Flavored, Mott's, ½ cup (123 g)	110	0	0	0	0	0
Apple Sauce, Bottled, Lite, Musselman's, ½ cup (122 g)	50	0	0	0	0	0
Apple Sauce, Bottled, Mott's, ½ cup (123 g)	100	0	0	0	0	0
Apple Sauce, Bottled, Natural, Unsweetened, No Preservatives, Mott's ½ cup (123 g)	50	0	0	0	0	0
Apple Sauce, Bottled, Raspberry, Mott's, 1 container (111 g)	90	0	0	0	0	0
Apple Sauce, Bottled, with Strawberries, Mott's, 1 container (111 g)	80	0	0	0	0	0
Apricot nectar, canned, 1 cup	140	tr	na	tr	na	0
Apricots, Canned, Heavy Syrup, Del Monte, ½ cup (127 g)	100	0	0	0	0	0
Apricots, Canned, Lite, Del Monte, ½ cup (122 g)	60	0	0	0	0	0
Apricots, dried, cooked, unsweetened, 1 cup	210	tr	na	tr	na	0
Apricots, dried, uncooked, 1 cup	310	1	3	tr	na	0
Apricots, raw, 3 apricots	50	tr	na	tr	na	0
Avocados, raw, whole, California, 1 avocado	305	28	83	5	15	0
Avocados, raw, whole, Florida, 1 avocado	340	23	61	5	13	0

FRUIT

FOOD/PORTION SIZE	CAL	FAT Total (g)	FAT As % of Cal	SAT FAT Total (g)	SAT FAT As % of Cal	CHOL (mg)
Bananas, raw, 1 banana	105	1	9	<1	<2	0
Blackberries, raw, 1 cup	75	1	12	<1	<2	0
Blueberries, Frozen, No Sugar Added, Seabrook Farms, ¾ cup (140 g)	70	0	0	0	0	0
Blueberries, frozen, sweetened, 10 oz	230	tr	na	tr	na	0
Blueberries, raw, 1 cup	80	1	11	tr	na	0
Cantaloupe, raw, ½ melon	95	1	9	<1	<1	0
Cherries, Canned, Bing, Pitted, In Heavy Syrup, Oregon Fruit Products, ½ cup (130 g)	110	0	0	0	0	0
Cherries, canned waterpack, sour, red, pitted, 1 cup	90	tr	na	<1	<1	0
Cherries, sweet, raw, 10 cherries	50	1	18	<1	<2	0
Cranberry Sauce, Canned, Jellied, Ocean Spray, ¼ cup (70 g)	110	0	0	0	0	0
Cranberry sauce, canned, sweetened, strained, 1 cup	420	tr	na	tr	na	0
Dates, Chopped, Amport Foods, ¼ cup (43 g)	135	0	0	0	0	0
Dates, Whole, Pitted, Amport Foods, ¼ cup, 7 dates	135	0	0	0	0	0
Figs, Calimyrna, Sun Dried, Sun-Maid, ¼ cup (40 g)	110	0	0	0	0	0
Figs, dried, 10 figs	475	2	4	<1	<1	0
Fruit, Mixed, Libby's Chunky, Lite, ½ cup (123 g)	60	0	0	0	0	0
Fruit Cocktail, Del Monte, ½ cup (127 g)	100	0	0	0	0	0
Fruit Cocktail, Del Monte Lite, ½ cup (124 g)	60	0	0	0	0	0
Fruit Cocktail, Libby's Lite, ½ cup (123 g)	60	0	0	0	0	0

FOOD/PORTION SIZE	CAL	FAT Total (g)	FAT As % of Cal	SAT FAT Total (g)	SAT FAT As % of Cal	CHOL (mg)
Grapefruit, canned, with syrup, 1 cup	150	tr	na	tr	na	0
Grapefruit, raw, ½ grapefruit	40	tr	na	tr	na	0
Grapes, Thompson seedless, 10 grapes	35	tr	na	<1	<3	0
Grapes, Tokay/Emperor, seeded, 10 grapes	40	tr	na	<1	<2	0
Honeydew melon, raw, ⅒ melon	45	tr	na	tr	na	0
Kiwifruit, raw, w/o skin, 1 kiwifruit	45	tr	na	tr	na	0
Lemons, raw, 1 lemon	15	tr	na	tr	na	0
Mangos, raw, 1 mango	135	1	7	<1	<1	0
Nectarines, raw, 1 nectarine	65	1	14	<1	<1	0
Olives, Bottled, Green, Stuffed, Spanish, Vlasic, 6 olives (16 g)	20	2	90	na	na	na
Olives, Canned, Black (ripe), Pitted, Early California, 3 olives (14 g)	25	2.5	90	0	0	0
Olives, ripe, mission, pitted, 3 small or 2 large	15	2	100	<1	<18	0
Oranges, raw, whole, w/o peel and seeds, 1 orange	60	tr	na	tr	na	0
Papayas, raw, ½-in. cubes, 1 cup	65	tr	na	<1	<1	0
Peaches, Canned, Yellow Cling, in Heavy Syrup, Del Monte, ½ cup (127 g)	100	0	0	0	0	0
Peaches, Canned, Yellow Cling, Lite, Del Monte, ½ cup (124 g)	60	0	0	0	0	0
Peaches, dried, uncooked, 1 cup	380	1	2	<1	<1	0
Peaches, Frozen, Seabrook Farms, ⅔ cup (140 g)	50	0	0	0	0	0
Peaches, raw, whole, 2½-in. diameter, 1 peach	35	tr	na	tr	na	0

FRUIT

FOOD/PORTION SIZE	CAL	FAT Total (g)	FAT As % of Cal	SAT FAT Total (g)	SAT FAT As % of Cal	CHOL (mg)
Peaches, Sliced, Natural Lite, Libby's, ½ cup (124 g)	60	0	0	0	0	0
Pears, Bartlett Canned, Heavy Syrup, Del Monte, ½ cup (127 g)	100	0	0	0	0	0
Pears, Bartlett Canned, Lite, Del Monte, ½ cup (124 g)	60	0	0	0	0	0
Pears, Bartlett raw, with skin, 1 pear	100	1	9	tr	na	0
Pears, Bosc raw, with skin, 1 pear	85	1	11	tr	na	0
Pears, D'Anjou raw, with skin, 1 pear	120	1	8	tr	na	0
Pears, Halves, Natural Lite, Libby's, ½ cup (124 g)	60	0	0	0	0	0
Pineapple, Canned, Clarified Pineapple Juice (all cuts), Dole, ½ cup (122 g)	60	0	0	0	0	0
Pineapple, Canned, Heavy Syrup (all cuts), Dole, ½ cup (123 g)	90	0	0	0	0	0
Pineapple, raw, diced, 1 cup	75	1	12	tr	na	0
Plums, canned, purple, juice pack, 3 plums	55	tr	na	tr	na	0
Plums, raw, 1½-in. diameter, 1 plum	15	tr	na	tr	na	0
Plums, raw, 2⅛-in. diameter, 1 plum	35	tr	na	tr	na	0
Prunes, dried, cooked, unsweetened, 1 cup	225	tr	na	tr	na	0
Prunes, Dried, Pitted, Dole, ¼ cup (40 g)	110	0	0	0	0	0
Prunes, dried, uncooked, 4 extra large or 5 large	115	tr	na	tr	na	0
Raisins, Seedless, Dole, ¼ cup (40 g)	130	0	0	0	0	0

FOOD/PORTION SIZE	CAL	FAT		SAT FAT		CHOL (mg)
		Total (g)	As % of Cal	Total (g)	As % of Cal	
Raspberries, Frozen, Seabrook Farms, ¾ cup (140 g)	130	0	0	0	0	0
Raspberries, in Syrup, Quick Thaw Pouch, Birds Eye, ½ cup (126 g)	90	0	0	0	0	0
Raspberries, raw, 1 cup	60	1	15	tr	na	0
Rhubarb, cooked, added sugar, 1 cup	280	tr	na	tr	na	0
Strawberries, Frozen, in Syrup, Quick Thaw Pouch, Birds Eye, ½ cup (134 g)	120	0	0	0	0	0
Strawberries, raw, whole, 1 cup	45	1	20	tr	na	0
Tangerine, canned, light syrup, 1 cup	155	tr	na	tr	na	0
Tangerine, raw, 2⅜-in. diameter, 1 tangerine	35	tr	na	tr	na	0
Watermelon, raw, diced, 1 cup	50	1	18	<1	<2	0
Watermelon, raw, 4 x 8-in. wedge, 1 piece	155	2	12	<1	<2	0

Gelatin, Pudding & Pie Filling

FOOD/PORTION SIZE	CAL	FAT		SAT FAT		CHOL (mg)
		Total (g)	As % of Cal	Total (g)	As % of Cal	
Custard, Americana, Jell-O, ¼ pkg (2 g)	80	0	0	0	0	0
Gelatin, All Flavors, Cups, Handi-Snacks, GELS, Kraft, 1 container (99 g)	80	0	0	0	0	0
Gelatin, All Flavors, Jell-O, ¼ pkg (22 g)	80	0	0	0	0	0

GELATIN, PUDDING & PIE FILLING

FOOD/PORTION SIZE	CAL	FAT Total (g)	FAT As % of Cal	SAT FAT Total (g)	SAT FAT As % of Cal	CHOL (mg)
Gelatin, All flavors, Sugar Free, Jell-O, ½ cup (average), ¼ pkg (25 g)	10	0	0	0	0	0
No Bake Dessert, Double Layer Banana, Made with Pudding, Jell-O, ⅛ pkg (37 g)	150	3.5	21	2	13	0
No Bake Dessert, Double Layer Chocolate, Made with Pudding, Jell-O, ⅛ pkg (41 g)	170	3.5	19	2.5	12	0
Pie Filling, Key Lime, Royal, Nabisco, dry mix for ⅙ filling for 8-in. pie (14 g)	50	0	0	0	0	0
Pudding, Cup, Chocolate, Del Monte, 1 container (99 g)	130	4	28	.5	3	0
Pudding, Cup, S'mores, Snack Pack Swirl, Hunts, 1 cup (99 g)	140	5	32	1.5	10	0
Pudding, Cup, Vanilla, Del Monte, 1 container (99 g)	120	3	23	.5	4	0
Pudding, Tapioca, Fat Free, Americana, Jell-O, ¼ pkg (23 g)	90	0	0	0	0	0
Pudding & Pie Filling, Banana Cream, Jell-O, ½ cup	90	0	0	0	0	0
Pudding & Pie Filling, Chocolate, Jell-O, ½ cup (25 g)	90	0	0	0	0	0
Pudding & Pie Filling, Chocolate Fudge, Jell-O, ½ cup (28 g)	100	0	0	0	0	0
Pudding & Pie Filling, Coconut Cream, Jell-O, ½ cup (25 g)	100	2	18	2	18	0
Pudding & Pie Filling, Cook & Serve, Lemon, Jell-O, ⅙ pkg (14 g)	50	0	0	0	0	0

GELATIN, PUDDING & PIE FILLING

FOOD/PORTION SIZE	CAL	FAT Total (g)	FAT As % of Cal	SAT FAT Total (g)	SAT FAT As % of Cal	CHOL (mg)
Pudding & Pie Filling, Cook & Serve, Vanilla, Fat Free, Jell-O Free, ¼ pkg (23 g)	90	0	0	0	0	0
Pudding & Pie Filling, Cook & Serve, Vanilla, Jell-O, ⅙ pkg (22 g)	80	0	0	0	0	0
Pudding & Pie Filling, Cook & Serve, Vanilla, Royal, ½ cup (21 g)	80	0	0	0	0	0
Pudding & Pie Filling, Instant, Butterscotch, Jell-O, ½ cup	90	0	0	0	0	0
Pudding & Pie Filling, Instant, Butterscotch, Sugar Free, Jell-O, ½ cup	70	0	0	0	0	0
Pudding & Pie Filling, Instant, Chocolate, Jell-O, ½ cup	100	0	0	0	0	0
Pudding & Pie Filling, Instant, Chocolate, Sugar Free, Jell-O, ½ cup	80	0	0	0	0	0
Pudding & Pie Filling, Instant, Chocolate Fudge, Jell-O, ¼ pkg (28 g)	100	0	0	0	0	0
Pudding & Pie Filling, Instant, Lemon, Jell-O, ¼ pkg (25 g)	90	0	0	0	0	0
Pudding & Pie Filling, Instant, Pistachio, Jell-O, ¼ pkg (25 g)	100	.5	5	0	0	0
Pudding & Pie Filling, Instant, Pistachio, Sugar Free, Jell-O, ¼ pkg (28 g)	30	0	0	0	0	0
Pudding & Pie Filling, Instant, French Vanilla, Jell-O, ¼ pkg (25 g)	90	0	0	0	0	0

GELATIN, PUDDING & PIE FILLING

FOOD/PORTION SIZE	CAL	FAT Total (g)	FAT As % of Cal	SAT FAT Total (g)	SAT FAT As % of Cal	CHOL (mg)
Pudding & Pie Filling, Instant, Vanilla, Jell-O, ¼ cup (25 g)	90	0	0	0	0	0
Pudding & Pie Filling, Instant, Vanilla, Sugar Free, Jell-O, ¼ cup (8 g)	25	0	0	0	0	0

Gravies & Sauces

FOOD/PORTION SIZE	CAL	FAT Total (g)	FAT As % of Cal	SAT FAT Total (g)	SAT FAT As % of Cal	CHOL (mg)
GRAVIES						
Beef, Bottled, Hearty, with Pieces of Beef, Pepperidge Farm, ¼ cup (60 ml)	25	1	36	0	0	<5
Beef, Canned, Franco-American, ¼ cup (60 ml)	30	2	60	1	30	<5
Brown, Bottled, Savory, Homestyle, Heinz, ¼ cup (60 g)	25	1	36	0	0	5
Brown, Dry Mix, Lawry's, 2 tbsp (6 g) for ¼ cup prepared	20	0	0	0	0	0
Chicken, Canned, Franco-American, ¼ cup (60 ml)	45	4	80	1	20	5
Chicken, Dry Mix, McCormick, ¼ pkg (6 g)	20	0	0	0	0	0
Chicken, Dry Mix, Swiss, 1 oz	89	.2	2	.1	1	0
Chicken, Golden, Bottled, with Pieces of Chicken, Pepperidge Farm, ¼ cup (60 g)	25	1	36	0	0	<5
Roasted Turkey, HomeStyle, Heinz, ¼ cup (60 g)	25	1	36	0	0	0

FOOD/PORTION SIZE	CAL	FAT		SAT FAT		CHOL (mg)
		Total (g)	As % of Cal	Total (g)	As % of Cal	
SAUCES						
Béarnaise Sauce Mix, Classic Sauces, Knorr, 1/5 pkg (5 g)	20	.5	23	0	0	0
Barbecue sauce, *see* BAKING PRODUCTS & CONDIMENTS						
Cheese, dry mix, prepared with milk, 1 cup	305	17	50	9	27	53
Hollandaise, prepared with water, 2 tbsp	30	3	90	2	60	7
Hollandaise Sauce Mix, Classic Sauces, Knorr, 1 tsp (2.5 g)	10	0	0	0	0	0
Picante Sauce, Mild, Pace, 2 tbsp (31.5 g)	10	0	0	0	0	0
Picante Sauce, Thick & Chunky, Mild, Old El Paso, 2 tbsp (30 g)	10	0	0	0	0	0
Soy sauce, *see* BAKING PRODUCTS & CONDIMENTS						
Spaghetti, Garden Combination, Chunky Garden Style, Ragu, 1/2 cup (128 g)	110	3.5	29	.5	4	0
Spaghetti, Garden Combination, Extra Chunky, Prego, 1/2 cup (120 ml)	90	1	10	.5	5	0
Spaghetti, Mushroom, Old World Style, Ragu, 1/2 cup (125 g)	80	3	34	.5	6	0
Spaghetti, Old World Style, Traditional, Ragu, 1/2 cup (125 g)	80	3	34	.5	6	0
Spaghetti, Sautéed Mushroom, Five Brothers, 1/2 cup (125 g)	70	3	39	.5	6	0

GRAVIES & SAUCES

FOOD/PORTION SIZE	CAL	FAT Total (g)	FAT As % of Cal	SAT FAT Total (g)	SAT FAT As % of Cal	CHOL (mg)
Spaghetti, Sautéed Onion & Mushroom, Hearty, Ragu, ½ cup (129 g)	110	3.5	29	.5	4	0
Spaghetti, with Fresh Mushrooms, Old World Style, Ragu, ½ cup (120 ml)	150	5	30	1.5	9	0
Spaghetti, with Meat, Prego, ½ cup (120 ml)	140	6	39	1.5	10	5
Spaghetti, Zesty Garlic & Cheese, Extra Chunky, Prego, ½ cup (120 ml)	130	3.5	24	1	7	0
White, Alfredo, Bottled, Five Brothers, ¼ cup (61 g)	110	10	82	6	49	40
White, Alfredo, Mix, Pasta Sauces, Knorr, 2 tbsp (15 g)	60	2.5	39	.5	8	5

Legumes & Nuts

FOOD/PORTION SIZE	CAL	FAT Total (g)	FAT As % of Cal	SAT FAT Total (g)	SAT FAT As % of Cal	CHOL (mg)
BEANS						
Black, Canned, Goya, ½ cup (122 g)	90	.5	5	0	0	0
Black, Dry, Goya, ¼ cup (38 g)	70	0	0	0	0	0
Chick Peas, Canned, Goya, ½ cup (122 g)	100	2	18	0	0	0
Chick Peas, Dry, Goya, ¼ cup (45 g)	110	2	16	0	0	0
Green, Canned, Cut, 50% less Sodium, Green Giant, ½ cup (120 g)	20	0	0	0	0	0
Green, Frozen, Cut, Green Giant, ¾ cup (78 g)	25	0	0	0	0	0

FOOD/PORTION SIZE	CAL	FAT Total (g)	FAT As % of Cal	SAT FAT Total (g)	SAT FAT As % of Cal	CHOL (mg)
Kidney, Canned, Red, Light, La Preferida, ½ cup (130 g)	120	1	8	0	0	0
Lentils, dry, cooked, 1 cup	215	1	4	<1	<1	0
Lentils, Dry, Jack Rabbit, ¼ cup (32 g)	70	0	0	0	0	0
Lima, Dry, Large, Jack Rabbit, ¼ cup (35 g)	70	0	0	0	0	0
Lima, immature seeds, frozen, cooked, drained: thin-seeded types (baby limas), 1 cup	188	1	5	<1	<1	0
Lima, immature seeds, frozen, cooked, drained: thick-seeded types (Fordhooks), 1 cup	170	1	5	<1	<1	0
Navy, Dry, Jack Rabbit, ¼ cup (38 g)	80	0	0	0	0	0
Pinto, Canned, Goya, ½ cup (126 g)	80	1	11	0	0	0
Pinto, Dry, Goya, ¼ cup (36 g)	60	0	0	0	0	0
Pork and Beans, Van Camp's, ½ cup (130 g)	110	<2	<12	<1	<4	0
Red Kidney, Canned, Goya, ½ cup (123 g)	90	1	10	0	0	0
Refried, Canned, Black, La Preferida, ½ cup (132 g)	120	0	0	0	0	0
Refried, Fat Free, Old El Paso, ½ cup (124 g)	110	0	0	0	0	0
Refried, Vegetarian, Old El Paso, ½ cup (118 g)	100	1	9	0	0	0
Snap, canned, drained, solids (cut), 1 cup	25	tr	na	tr	na	0
Snap, cooked, drained, from frozen (cut), 1 cup	35	tr	na	tr	na	0
Snap, cooked, drained, from raw (cut and French style), 1 cup	45	tr	na	<1	<2	0

LEGUMES & NUTS

FOOD/PORTION SIZE	CAL	FAT Total (g)	FAT As % of Cal	SAT FAT Total (g)	SAT FAT As % of Cal	CHOL (mg)
Sprouts (mung), raw, 1 cup	30	tr	na	tr	na	0
Tahini, 1 tbsp	95	7	66	1	9	0
White, with sliced frankfurters, canned, 1 cup	365	18	44	7	17	30

NUTS

FOOD/PORTION SIZE	CAL	FAT Total (g)	FAT As % of Cal	SAT FAT Total (g)	SAT FAT As % of Cal	CHOL (mg)
Almonds, Shelled, Whole, Evon's, 1 oz (28 g)	170	13	69	1	5	0
Almonds, Sliced, Evon's, 1 oz (28 g)	170	13	69	1	5	0
Brazil, shelled, 1 oz	185	19	92	4	19	0
Cashew, Halves, Lightly Salted, Planters, 1 oz (28 g)	160	13	73	2.5	14	0
Cashew, Halves, Salted, Planters, 1 oz (28 g)	170	14	74	2.5	13	0
Cashew, salted, roasted in oil, 1 cup	869	67	69	14	14	0
Chestnuts, European, roasted, shelled, 1 cup	350	3	8	tr	na	0
Coconut, raw, piece, 1.6 oz (45 g)	160	15	84	13	73	0
Filberts (Hazelnuts), Evon's, 1 oz (28 g)	180	16	80	1	5	0
Macadamia, Salted, Mauna Loa, 1 oz (28 g)	200	21	95	3	14	0
Macadamia, salted, roasted in oil, 1 cup	1088	103	85	16	13	0
Mixed, Deluxe, Planters, 1 oz (28 g)	170	16	85	2	11	0
Mixed, Lightly Salted, Planters, 1 oz (28 g)	170	15	79	2	11	0
Peanut Butter, Creamy, Skippy, 2 tbsp (32 g)	190	17	81	3.5	17	0
Peanut Butter, Extra Crunchy, Jif, 2 tbsp (32 g)	190	16	76	3	14	0

FOOD/PORTION SIZE	CAL.	FAT		SAT. FAT		CHOL. (mg)
		Total (g)	As % of Cal.	Total (g)	As % of Cal.	
Peanuts, Cocktail, Salted, Planters, 1 oz (28 g)	170	14	74	2	11	0
Peanuts, Dry Roasted, Planter's, about 39 peanuts, 1 oz (28 g)	160	13	73	2	11	0
Peanuts, salted, roasted in oil, 1 cup	869	64	66	9	9	0
Pecans, Halves, Evon's, 1 oz (28 g)	200	20	90	2	9	0
Pistachio, dried, shelled, 1 oz	165	13	71	2	11	0
Walnuts, Black, Chopped, Evon's, 1 oz (28 g)	190	17	81	1.5	7	0
Walnuts, Chopped, Evon's, 1 oz (28 g)	200	20	90	1.5	7	0
PEAS						
Black Eyed, Dry, Jack Rabbit, ¼ cup (37 g)	90	0	0	0	0	0
Green Split, Dry, Goya, ¼ cup (45 g)	110	0	0	0	0	0
Split, dry, cooked, 1 cup	230	1	4	<1	<1	0
Yellow Split, Dry, Jack Rabbit, ¼ cup (45g)	110	0	0	0	0	0
SEEDS						
Pumpkin, Roasted and Salted, David, (50 g)	320	25	70	5	14	0
Pumpkin/squash kernels, dry, hulled, 1 oz	155	13	75	2	12	0
Sesame, dry, hulled, 1 tbsp	45	4	80	<1	<12	0
Sunflower, dry, hulled, 1 oz	160	14	79	<2	<8	0
Sunflower, Roasted and Salted, David, ¼ cup (30 g)	190	15	71	1.5	7	0
SOY PRODUCTS						
Miso, 1 cup	568	14	22	2	3	0

LEGUMES & NUTS

FOOD/PORTION SIZE	CAL	FAT Total (g)	FAT As % of Cal	SAT FAT Total (g)	SAT FAT As % of Cal	CHOL (mg)
Soybeans, dry, cooked, drained, 1 cup	298	13	39	2	6	0
Tofu, Firm, Nasoya, 1/5 block	80	4	45	.5	6	0

Meats

FOOD/PORTION SIZE	CAL	FAT Total (g)	FAT As % of Cal	SAT FAT Total (g)	SAT FAT As % of Cal	CHOL (mg)
BEEF						
Chipped, dried, 2½ oz	118	3	23	1	8	50
Chuck blade, lean only, braised/simmered/pot roasted, approx. 2¼ oz	168	9	48	4	21	66
Corned, Canned, Hereford, 2 oz (56 g)	130	7	48	3	21	50
Corned, Lean, Carl Buddig, 1 pack (71 g)	100	5	45	2	18	0
Dried, Extra Lean, Hormel, 10 slices (28 g)	50	1.5	27	.5	9	25
Ground, patty, broiled, regular, 3 oz	245	18	66	7	26	76
Ground, patty, lean, broiled, 3 oz	230	16	63	6	27	74
Heart, lean, braised, 3 oz	150	5	30	2	12	164
Liver, fried, 3 oz	185	7	34	3	15	410
Roast, eye of round, lean only, oven cooked, approx. 2½ oz	135	5	33	2	13	52
Roast, rib, lean only, oven cooked, approx. 2¼ oz	150	9	54	4	24	49
Round, bottom, lean only, braised/simmered/pot roasted, 24.5 oz	175	8	41	3	15	75
Steak, sirloin, lean only, broiled, 2½ oz	150	6	36	3	18	64

FOOD/PORTION SIZE	CAL	FAT Total (g)	FAT As % of Cal	SAT FAT Total (g)	SAT FAT As % of Cal	CHOL (mg)
FRANKS & SAUSAGES						
Corn Dogs, Ball Park, 1 dog (75 g)	220	13	53	3	12	20
Franks, Beef, Jumbo, Eckrich, 1 frank (57 g)	190	17	81	8	38	35
Franks, Beef, Oscar Mayer, 1 link (45 g)	140	13	84	6	39	25
Franks, Fun, Ball Park, 2 franks (112 g)	350	21	54	6	15	45
Franks, Turkey, Butterball, 1 frank (45 g)	100	8	72	<4	<32	35
Franks, Turkey/Pork/Beef, Jumbo, Low Fat, Healthy Choice, 1 frank (57 g)	70	1.5	19	.5	6	30
Sausage, Pork, Links, Tennessee Pride, 3 cooked links (42 g)	140	12	77	4	26	30
Sausage, Pork, Regular, Jimmy Dean, 2 oz cooked (56 g)	250	24	86	8	30	50
Sausage, Turkey/Pork/Beef, Brown 'N Serve, Original, Swift Premium, 2 links (45 g)	150	14	84	5	30	35
Weiners, Oscar Mayer, 1 link (45 g)	150	13	78	5	30	30
GAME						
Buffalo, roasted, 3 oz	111	2	16	<1	na	52
Venison, roasted, 3 oz	134	3	20	1	7	95
LAMB						
Chops, shoulder, lean only, braised, approx. 1¾ oz	135	7	47	3	20	44
Leg, lean only, roasted, approx. 2⅔ oz	140	6	39	3	19	65

MEATS

FOOD/PORTION SIZE	CAL	FAT Total (g)	FAT As % of Cal	SAT FAT Total (g)	SAT FAT As % of Cal	CHOL (mg)
Loin, chop, lean only, broiled, approx. 2⅓ oz	182	10	49	4	20	60
Rib, lean only, roasted, 2 oz	130	7	48	4	28	50
LUNCHEON MEATS						
Bologna, Beef, Oscar Mayer, 1 slice (28 g)	90	8	80	4	40	15
Bologna, Lite, Oscar Mayer, 1 slice (28 g)	60	4	60	1.5	23	15
Bologna, Oscar Mayer, 1 slice (28 g)	90	8	80	3	30	30
Braunschweiger Sausage, Oscar Mayer, 2 oz (56 g)	190	17	81	6	28	90
Chicken, roll, light, 2 oz	90	4	40	1	10	28
Ham, Baked, Low Fat, Healthy Choice, 1 slice (28 g)	30	1	30	.5	15	15
Ham, Boiled, Oscar Mayer, 3 slices (56 g)	60	2	30	1	15	30
Ham, Chopped, Oscar Mayer, 1 slice (28 g)	50	3	18	1	6	15
Ham, extra lean, cooked, 2 slices, 2 oz	75	3	36	1	12	27
Ham, regular, cooked, 2 slices, 2 oz	105	6	51	2	17	32
Ham, Smoked, Deli Select, Hillshire Farm, 6 slices (57 g)	60	1.5	23	.5	8	25
Pork, Canned Lunch Meat, SPAM, 2 oz (56 g)	170	16	85	6	32	40
Salami, Hard, Oscar Mayer, 3 slices (27 g)	100	9	81	3	27	25
Salami sausage, cooked, 2 oz	141	11	70	5	32	37
Salami sausage, dry, 12-slice pack, 2 slices, ⅔ oz	84	6	64	2	21	16

FOOD/PORTION SIZE	CAL	FAT Total (g)	FAT As % of Cal	SAT FAT Total (g)	SAT FAT As % of Cal	CHOL (mg)
Sandwich spread, beef/pork, 1 tbsp	35	3	77	<1	<23	6
Sandwich Spread, Ham & Pork, Deviled Ham, Underwood, ¼ cup (56 g)	160	14	79	4.5	25	45
Turkey, Breast, Healthy Choice, 6 slices, (54 g)	60	<2	<23	<1	<8	25
Turkey, Breast, Roasted, Oscar Mayer, 1 slice (28 g)	30	1	30	0	0	0
Turkey, thigh meat, ham cured, 2 oz	75	3	36	1	12	32
Turkey Bologna, Louis Rich Turkey Cold Cuts, 1 slice (28 g)	50	4	72	1	18	20
Turkey Ham, Breast, Hickory Smoked, Louis Rich 1 slice (28 g)	25	0	0	0	0	10
Turkey Ham, Thigh Meat, Louis Rich, 3 slices (63 g)	70	2	26	.5	6	45
Turkey Salami, Louis Rich, 1 slice (28 g)	40	2.5	56	1	23	20
Vienna Sausage, Hormel, 2 oz (56 g)	150	14	84	5	30	45
PORK						
Bacon, Canadian, Roses, 3 slices cooked, (62 g)	60	1.5	23	.5	8	25
Bacon, Oscar Mayer, 2 slices cooked, (12 g)	60	5	75	1.5	23	10
Chop, loin, fresh, lean only, broiled, 2½ oz	163	7	39	3	17	69
Chop, loin, fresh, lean only, pan fried, approx. 2½ oz	181	10	50	4	20	73
Ham, Boiled, Oscar Mayer, 3 slices (63 g)	60	2	30	1	15	30
Ham, canned, roasted, 3 oz	140	7	45	2	13	35

MEATS

FOOD/PORTION SIZE	CAL	FAT Total (g)	FAT As % of Cal	SAT FAT Total (g)	SAT FAT As % of Cal	CHOL (mg)
Ham, leg, fresh, lean only, roasted, 2½ oz	156	8	46	3	17	67
Ham, light cure, lean only, roasted, approx. 2½ oz	107	4	34	1	8	38
Rib, fresh, lean only, roasted, 2½ oz	173	8	42	3	16	56
Shoulder cut, fresh, lean only, braised, 2²/₅ oz	169	8	43	3	16	78
Tenderloin, roasted, lean, 3 oz	139	4	26	1	6	67
Turkey Bacon, Louis Rich, 1 slice (14 g)	30	<3	75	<1	<15	10

VEAL

FOOD/PORTION SIZE	CAL	FAT Total (g)	FAT As % of Cal	SAT FAT Total (g)	SAT FAT As % of Cal	CHOL (mg)
Cubed, lean only, braised, 3½ oz	188	4	19	1	5	145
Cutlet, leg, lean only, braised, 3½ oz	203	6	27	2	9	135
Rib, lean only, roasted, 3½ oz	177	7	36	2	10	115

Packaged Entrées

FOOD/PORTION SIZE	CAL	FAT Total (g)	FAT As % of Cal	SAT FAT Total (g)	SAT FAT As % of Cal	CHOL (mg)
Beefaroni, Chef Boyardee, 1 cup (249 g)	260	7	24	3	10	25
Beef Pasta, Hamburger Helper, Betty Crocker, ⅔ cup mix	120	1	8	0	0	0
Beef Stew, Dinty Moore, 1 cup (236 g)	230	14	55	7	27	40
Cheeseburger Macaroni, Hamburger Helper, ⅓ cup mix	180	5	25	1.5	8	5

FOOD/PORTION SIZE	CAL	FAT Total (g)	FAT As % of Cal	SAT FAT Total (g)	SAT FAT As % of Cal	CHOL (mg)
Chicken, Sweet & Sour, LaChoy, 1 cup (254 g)	160	2.5	14	1	6	25
Chili, Turkey, with Beans, Hormel, 1 cup (247 g)	200	3	13.5	1	4.5	50
Chili, with Beans, Hormel, 1 cup (247 g)	340	17	45	7	19	60
Chili con carne, with beans, canned, 1 cup	286	13	41	6	19	43
Chow Mein, Beef, LaChoy, 1 cup (247 g)	110	1.5	12	1	8	10
Chow Mein, Chicken, LaChoy, 1 cup (250 g)	110	4.5	37	1	8	10
Lasagna, Hamburger Helper, ⅔ cup mix	140	1	6	0	0	0
Macaroni and Cheese Deluxe Dinner, Kraft, about 1 cup (98 g)	320	10	28	6	17	25
Macaroni and Cheese Dinner, Original, Kraft, about 1 cup (70 g)	260	3	9	1	3	10
Shells and Cheese, Original, Velveeta, Kraft, 1 cup (126 g)	360	13	33	8	20	40
Spaghetti, Canned, in Tomato Sauce with Cheese, Franco-American, 1 cup (252 g)	210	2	9	1	4	5
Spaghetti, with Meatballs, Franco-American, 1 cup (252 g)	270	10	33	5	17	30
Spaghetti Dinner, Mild American Style, Kraft, prepared, about 1 cup (230 g)	270	<5	<15	1	3	<5
Spaghetti Dinner, Tangy Italian Style, Kraft, about 1 cup (56 g)	270	3	10	<1	<2	5
SpaghettiO's, with Meatballs, Franco-American, 1 cup (252 g)	260	11	38	5	17	20

PACKAGED ENTRÉES

FOOD/PORTION SIZE	CAL	FAT Total (g)	FAT As % of Cal	SAT FAT Total (g)	SAT FAT As % of Cal	CHOL (mg)
Ravioli, in Tomato & Meat Sauce, Beef, Chef Boyardee, 1 cup (244 g)	230	5	20	2.5	10	20

Pasta

FOOD/PORTION SIZE	CAL	FAT Total (g)	FAT As % of Cal	SAT FAT Total (g)	SAT FAT As % of Cal	CHOL (mg)
Angel Hair, Prince, 2 oz (56 g)	210	1	4	0	0	0
Egg Noodles Substitute, Cholesterol Free, No Yolks, 2 oz dry (56 g)	210	<1	<2	0	0	0
Linguine, Creamette, 2 oz (56 g)	210	1	4	0	0	0
Macaroni, Elbow, Creamette, ½ cup (56 g)	210	1	4	0	0	0
Macaroni, enriched, cooked, tender, hot, 1 cup	155	1	6	<1	<1	0
Macaroni and cheese dishes, see PACKAGED ENTRÉES						
Noodles, chow mein, canned, 1 cup	220	11	45	2	8	5
Noodles, Chow Mein, China Boy, ½ cup (25 g)	125	5	36	1	7	0
Noodles, egg, enriched, cooked, 1 cup	200	2	9	1	5	50
Noodles, Egg, Extra Broad, Mrs. Grass, 1½ cups (56 g)	210	2.5	11	1	4	55
Spaghetti, Creamette, 2 oz (56 g)	210	1	4	0	0	0
Spaghetti, enriched, cooked, firm, hot, 1 cup	190	1	5	<1	<1	0

FOOD/PORTION SIZE	CAL	FAT Total (g)	FAT As % of Cal	SAT FAT Total (g)	SAT FAT As % of Cal	CHOL (mg)
Spaghetti, Enriched No. 3, Prince, 2 oz (56 g)	210	1	4	0	0	0
Spaghetti, with sauce/meat, *see* PACKAGED ENTRÉES						
Vermicelli, Creamette, 2 oz (dry)	210	1	4	0	0	0

Poultry

FOOD/PORTION SIZE	CAL	FAT Total (g)	FAT As % of Cal	SAT FAT Total (g)	SAT FAT As % of Cal	CHOL (mg)
Chicken, boneless, canned, 5 oz	235	11	42	3	11	88
Chicken, breast, flesh only, roasted, 3 oz	140	3	19	<1	<6	73
Chicken, broiler-fryer, breast, w/o skin, roasted, 3½ oz	165	4	22	1	5	85
Chicken, drumstick, roasted, approx. 1³/₅ oz	75	2	24	<1	<8	26
Chicken, light and dark meat, flesh only, stewed, 1 cup	332	17	46	1	3	117
Chicken, liver, cooked, 1 liver	30	1	30	<1	<12	120
Chicken, white and dark meat, w/o skin, roasted, 3½ oz	190	7	33	2	9	89
Cold cuts, chicken or turkey, *see* LUNCHEON MEATS *in* MEATS *section*						
Duck, flesh only, roast, ½ duck, approx. 7¾ oz	445	24	49	11	22	197
Frankfurters, chicken or turkey, *see* FRANKS & SAUSAGES *in* MEATS *section*						

POULTRY

FOOD/PORTION SIZE	CAL	FAT Total (g)	FAT As % of Cal	SAT FAT Total (g)	SAT FAT As % of Cal	CHOL (mg)
Turkey, dark meat only, w/o skin, roasted, 3½ oz	187	7	34	2	10	85
Turkey, flesh only, 1 light and 2 dark slices, 3 oz (85 g)	145	4	25	1	6	65
Turkey, flesh only, light and dark meat, chopped or diced, roasted, 1 cup, 5 oz (140 g)	240	7	26	2	8	106
Turkey, flesh only, light meat, roasted, 2 pieces, 3 oz (85 g)	135	3	20	1	7	59
Turkey, frozen, boneless, light and dark meat, seasoned, chunked, roasted, 3 oz	130	5	35	2	14	45
Turkey, patties, breaded, battered, fried, 1 patty	180	12	60	3	15	40
Turkey, white meat only, w/o skin, roasted, 3½ oz	157	3	17	1	6	69
Turkey and gravy, frozen, 5 oz pkg	95	3	28	1	9	18

Rice

FOOD/PORTION SIZE	CAL	FAT Total (g)	FAT As % of Cal	SAT FAT Total (g)	SAT FAT As % of Cal	CHOL (mg)
Beef, Rice & Sauce, Lipton, Mix, ½ cup (63 g)	230	1	4	0	0	0
Beef Flavor, Rice-A-Roni, Mix, 2.5 oz (70 g)	240	1.5	6	0	0	0
Broccoli auGratin, Country Inn, Uncle Ben's, 2 oz (56 g)	200	2	9	1	5	5
Brown, Instant, Whole Grain, Minute Brand, ½ cup cooked (43 g)	170	1.5	8	na	na	na

FOOD/PORTION SIZE	CAL	FAT Total (g)	FAT As % of Cal	SAT FAT Total (g)	SAT FAT As % of Cal	CHOL (mg)
Brown & Wild Mushroom Recipe, Uncle Ben's, 1 cup cooked, 2 oz (56 g)	190	1.5	7	0	0	0
Chicken, Rice-A-Roni, Mix, 1 cup prepared, 2.5 oz (70 g)	240	1	4	0	0	0
Chicken & Broccoli, Golden Sauté, Lipton, Mix, 1/2 cup (65 g)	260	4.5	16	1.5	5	0
Chicken & Broccoli, Rice-A-Roni, Mix, 2.5 oz (70 g)	240	1.5	6	0	0	0
Extra-Long Grain, Riceland, 1/4 cup (45 g)	160	0	0	0	0	0
Instant, ready-to-serve, hot, 1 cup	180	0	0	0	0	0
Instant, Uncle Ben's, 1/2 cup (52 g)	190	.5	2	0	0	0
Long Grain, Converted, Uncle Ben's, 1/4 cup (49 g)	170	0	0	0	0	0
Long Grain & Wild, Original Recipe, Uncle Ben's, 2 oz (56 g)	190	.5	2	0	0	0
Long Grain & Wild, Original, Rice-A-Roni, Mix, 2 oz (56 g)	190	.5	2	0	0	0
Mushroom, Rice & Sauce, Lipton, Mix, 1/2 cup (63 g)	220	1	4	1	4	0
Oriental Stir Fry, Rice-A-Roni, Mix, 2.5 oz (70 g)	240	1	4	0	0	0
Parboiled, cooked, hot, 1 cup	185	tr	na	tr	na	0
Parboiled, raw, 1 cup	685	1	1	<1	<1	0
Rice Pilaf, Rice-A-Roni, Mix, 2.5 oz (70 g)	240	1	4	0	0	0
Spanish Fiesta, Golden Sauté, Lipton, Mix, 1/2 cup (65 g)	250	4.5	16	1.5	5	0

RICE

FOOD/PORTION SIZE	CAL.	FAT Total (g)	FAT As % of Cal.	SAT. FAT Total (g)	SAT. FAT As % of Cal.	CHOL. (mg)
White, enriched, cooked, hot, 1 cup	225	tr	na	<1	<1	0
White, Extra Long Grain, Riceland, ¼ cup (45 g)	160	0	0	0	0	0
White, Instant, Minute Rice, ½ cup (44 g)	170	0	0	0	0	0
White, Long Grain, Boil-in-Bag, Minute Rice, ½ bag (50 g)	190	0	0	0	0	0

Salad Dressings

FOOD/PORTION SIZE	CAL	FAT Total (g)	FAT As % of Cal	SAT FAT Total (g)	SAT FAT As % of Cal	CHOL (mg)
Blue Cheese, Chunky, Fat Free, Wishbone, 2 tbsp (30 ml)	30	0	0	0	0	0
Blue Cheese, Chunky, Lite, Wishbone, 2 tbsp (30 ml)	80	7	79	1.5	17	0
Blue Cheese, Chunky, Lite & Luscious, Refrigerated, Marie's, 2 tbsp (30 ml)	100	7	63	.5	5	5
Blue Cheese, Chunky, Refrigerated, Marie's, 2 tbsp (30 ml)	180	19	95	3.5	18	15
Blue Cheese, Chunky, Wishbone, 2 tbsp (30 ml)	170	17	90	3	16	10
Blue Cheese, Fat Free, Hidden Valley, 2 tbsp (32 ml)	20	0	0	0	0	0
Blue Cheese Flavor, Fat Free Dressing, Kraft, 2 tbsp (34 g)	50	0	0	0	0	0
Caesar, Classic, Seven Seas, 2 tbsp (31 g)	100	10	90	1.5	14	0
Caesar, Creamy, Refrigerated, Marie's, 2 tbsp (30 ml)	180	18	90	3	15	20

FOOD/PORTION SIZE	CAL	FAT		SAT FAT		CHOL (mg)
		Total (g)	As % of Cal	Total (g)	As % of Cal	
Caesar, Dry Mix, Good Seasons, 2 tbsp prepared	150	16	96	2.5	15	0
Caesar, Fat Free, Wishbone, 2 tbsp (30 ml)	30	0	0	0	0	0
Caesar, Hidden Valley, 2 tbsp (30 g)	110	11	90	1	8	5
Caesar, Wishbone, 2 tbsp (30 ml)	110	10	82	2	16	15
Catalina, Fat Free Dressing, Kraft, 2 tbsp (33 g)	35	0	0	0	0	0
Catalina, Kraft, 2 tbsp (32 g)	120	10	75	1.5	11	0
Catalina, with Honey, Kraft, 2 tbsp (32 g)	140	12	77	2	13	0
Coleslaw, Hellman's, 2 tbsp (30 g)	110	10	82	1.5	12	0
French, Deluxe, Fat Free, Wishbone, 2 tbsp (30 ml)	30	0	0	0	0	0
French, Deluxe, Wishbone, 2 tbsp (30 ml)	120	11	83	1.5	11	0
French, Fat Free Dressing, Kraft, 2 tbsp (35 g)	50	0	0	0	0	0
French, Honey, Dry Mix, Good Seasons, ⅛ envelope, 2 tbsp prepared (6 g)	160	15	84	2	11	0
French, Honey, Refrigerated, T. Marzetti, 2 tbsp (33 g)	160	14	79	2	11	0
French, Kraft, 2 tbsp (31 g)	120	12	90	2	15	0
French, Sweet 'N Spicy, Fat Free, Wishbone, 2 tbsp (30 ml)	30	0	0	0	0	0
French, Sweet 'N Spicy, Wishbone, 2 tbsp (30 ml)	130	12	83	2	14	0
Garlic, Creamy, Italian, Refrigerated, Marie's, 2 tbsp (30 ml)	180	19	95	3	15	15
Garlic, Creamy, Kraft, 2 tbsp (30 g)	110	11	90	2	16	0

SALAD DRESSINGS

FOOD/PORTION SIZE	CAL.	FAT Total (g)	FAT As % of Cal.	SAT. FAT Total (g)	SAT. FAT As % of Cal.	CHOL. (mg)
Garlic, Creamy Roasted, Fat Free, Wishbone, 2 tbsp (30 ml)	40	0	0	0	0	0
Garlic & Herb, Dry Mix, Good Seasons, 2 tbsp prepared	140	15	96	2	13	0
Greco, Special Edition, Classic Dressing, Lawry's, 2 tbsp (30 ml)	130	13	90	2	14	0
Green Goddess, Seven Seas, 2 tbsp (31 g)	120	13	98	2	15	0
Herb, Zesty, Dry Mix, Fat Free, Good Seasons, ⅛ envelope, 2 tbsp prepared (3 g)	10	0	0	0	0	0
Honey Dijon, Fat Free Dressing, Kraft, 2 tbsp (34 g)	50	0	0	0	0	0
Italian, Classic Dressing, Lawry's, 2 tbsp (30 ml)	140	14	90	2.5	16	5
Italian, Creamy, Fat Free Dressing, Kraft, 2 tbsp (34 g)	50	0	0	0	0	0
Italian, Creamy, Wishbone, 2 tbsp (30 ml)	110	10	82	2	16	0
Italian, Dry Mix, Good Seasons, 2 tbsp prepared	140	15	96	2	13	0
Italian, Fat Free, Seven Seas, 2 tbsp (32 g)	10	0	0	0	0	0
Italian, Fat Free Dressing, Kraft, 2 tbsp (31 g)	15	0	0	0	0	0
Italian, House, with Olive Oil, Kraft, 2 tbsp (30 g)	120	12	90	2	15	<5
Italian, ⅓ Less Fat, Seven Seas, 2 tbsp (31 g)	45	4	80	.5	10	0
Italian, Lite, Wishbone, 2 tbsp (30 ml)	15	.5	30	0	0	0
Italian, Mild, Dry Mix, Good Seasons, 2 tbsp prepared	150	15	90	2.5	15	0

FOOD/PORTION SIZE	CAL.	FAT		SAT. FAT		CHOL. (mg)
		Total (g)	As % of Cal.	Total (g)	As % of Cal.	
Italian, Parmesan, Dry Mix, Good Seasons, ⅛ envelope, 2 tbsp prepared (6 g)	150	16	96	2.5	15	0
Italian, Robusto, Wishbone, 2 tbsp (30 ml)	100	9	81	1.5	14	0
Italian, Seven Seas, 2 tbsp (31 g)	90	9	90	1.5	15	0
Italian, Tomato & Herb, Kraft, 2 tbsp (31 g)	100	10	90	1.5	14	0
Italian, Wishbone, 2 tbsp (30 ml)	100	9	81	1.5	14	0
Italian, Zesty, Dry Mix, Good Seasons, 2 tbsp prepared	140	15	96	2	13	0
Lemon Pepper, Classic Dressing, Lawry's, 2 tbsp (30 ml)	130	13	90	2	14	0
Miracle Whip, Light Dressing, Kraft, 1 tbsp (16 g)	35	3	77	0	0	<5
Miracle Whip, Nonfat, Kraft Free, 1 tbsp (16 g)	15	0	0	0	0	0
Miracle Whip, Original, Kraft, 1 tbsp (15 g)	70	7	90	1	13	5
Oriental Sesame, Dry Mix, Good Seasons, 2 tbsp prepared	150	16	96	2.5	15	0
Original, Buttermilk Recipe, Dry Mix, Hidden Valley, 2 tbsp (30 g)	0	0	0	0	0	0
Original, Dry Mix, Hidden Valley, 2 tbsp (30 g)	5	0	0	0	0	0
Parmesan, Italian, Fat Free, Hidden Valley, 2 tbsp (32 g)	20	0	0	0	0	0
Parmesan, Italian, Hidden Valley, 2 tbsp (30 g)	110	11	90	1	8	0

SALAD DRESSINGS

FOOD/PORTION SIZE	CAL	FAT Total (g)	FAT As % of Cal	SAT FAT Total (g)	SAT FAT As % of Cal	CHOL (mg)
Peppercorn, Parmesan, Refrigerated, T. Marzetti, 2 tbsp (29 g)	170	18	95	2.5	13	10
Poppyseed, Refrigerated, T. Marzetti, 2 tbsp (32 g)	140	11	71	1.5	10	10
Potato Salad, Hellman's, 2 tbsp (30 g)	110	11	90	1.5	12	0
Ranch, Caesar, Kraft, 2 tbsp (30 g)	110	11	90	2	16	10
Ranch, Creamy, Refrigerated, Marie's, 2 tbsp (30 ml)	190	20	95	3	14	15
Ranch, Cucumber, Kraft, 2 tbsp (30 g)	140	15	96	2	13	0
Ranch, Fat Free, Seven Seas, 2 tbsp (35 g)	50	0	0	0	0	0
Ranch, Fat Free, Wishbone, 2 tbsp (30 ml)	40	0	0	0	0	0
Ranch, Garlic!, Hidden Valley, 2 tbsp (30 g)	130	13	90	1.5	10	5
Ranch, Kraft, 2 tbsp (29 g)	170	18	95	3	16	10
Ranch, ⅓ Less Fat, Kraft, 2 tbsp (30 g)	110	11	90	2	16	10
Ranch, Lite, Wishbone, 2 tbsp (30 ml)	100	9	81	2	18	5
Ranch, Original, Fat Free, Hidden Valley, 2 tbsp (32 g)	45	0	0	0	0	0
Ranch, Original, Hidden Valley, 2 tbsp (30 g)	140	14	90	1.5	10	10
Ranch, Peppercorn, Fat Free, Hidden Valley, 2 tbsp (32 g)	30	0	0	0	0	0
Ranch, Peppercorn, Kraft, 2 tbsp (29 g)	170	18	95	3	16	10
Ranch, Sour Cream & Onion, Fat Free Dressing, Kraft, 2 tbsp (35 g)	45	0	0	0	0	0
Ranch, with Bacon, Hidden Valley, 2 tbsp (29 g)	150	15	90	1.5	9	10

FOOD/PORTION SIZE	CAL	FAT Total (g)	FAT As % of Cal	SAT FAT Total (g)	SAT FAT As % of Cal	CHOL (mg)
Ranchero, Special Edition, Classic Dressing, Lawry's, 2 tbsp (30 ml)	120	12	90	2	15	0
Russian, Kraft, 2 tbsp (33 g)	130	10	70	1.5	10	0
Russian, Wishbone, 2 tbsp (30 ml)	110	6	49	1	8	0
San Francisco, Special Edition, Classic Dressing, Lawry's, 2 tbsp (30 ml)	140	13	84	2	13	0
Slaw, Refrigerated, T. Marzetti, 2 tbsp (31 g)	170	16	85	2.5	13	30
Sour Cream & Dill, Refrigerated, Marie's, 2 tbsp (30 ml)	190	20	95	3	14	15
Thousand Island, Fat Free Dressing, Kraft, 2 tbsp (33 g)	40	0	0	0	0	0
Thousand Island, Kraft, 2 tbsp (31 g)	120	10	75	1.5	11	10
Thousand Island, ⅓ Less Fat, Kraft, 2 tbsp (32 g)	70	4.5	58	.5	6	5
Thousand Island, Refrigerated, Marie's, 2 tbsp (30 ml)	160	15	84	2.5	14	15
Thousand Island, Wishbone, 2 tbsp (30 ml)	130	12	83	2	14	10
Tuna Salad, Hellman's, 2 tbsp (27 g)	90	9	90	1.5	15	0
Vegetable Dip & Dressing, Refrigerated, T. Marzetti, 2 tbsp (28 g)	170	18	95	2.5	13	3
Vinaigrette, Red Wine, Classic Dressing, Lawry's, 2 tbsp (30 ml)	90	7	70	1	10	0
Vinaigrette, Red Wine, Wishbone, 2 tbsp (30ml)	80	5	56	1	11	0
Vinaigrette, White Wine, Classic Dressing, Lawry's, 2 tbsp (30 ml)	130	14	97	2	14	0

SALAD DRESSINGS

FOOD/PORTION SIZE	CAL	FAT Total (g)	FAT As % of Cal	SAT FAT Total (g)	SAT FAT As % of Cal	CHOL (mg)
Vinegar, Red Wine, Fat Free Dressing, Kraft, 2 tbsp (32 g)	15	0	0	0	0	0
Vinegar & Oil, Red Wine, Seven Seas, 2 tbsp (31 g)	90	9	90	1.5	15	0

Snacks

FOOD/PORTION SIZE	CAL	FAT Total (g)	FAT As % of Cal	SAT FAT Total (g)	SAT FAT As % of Cal	CHOL (mg)
CORN CHIPS						
Bugles, 1⅓ cups (30 g)	160	9	51	8	45	0
Doritos, Cooler Ranch, about 12 chips, 1 oz (28 g)	140	7	45	1	6	0
Doritos, Nacho Cheesier, about 11 chips, 1 oz (28 g)	140	7	45	1	6	0
Fritos Corn Chips, about 32 chips, 1 oz (28 g)	160	10	56	<2	<8	0
Tortilla Chips, No Oil, No Salt, All Natural, California Bakes, Garden of Eatin', about 12 chips, 1 oz (28 g)	110	1	8	0	0	0
Tostitos, 100% White Corn Restaurant Style, about 6 chips, 1 oz (28 g)	130	6	42	1	7	0
DIPS						
Avocado, Deans, 2 tbsp (31 g)	60	5	75	1	15	0
Bean Dip, Frito-Lay's, 2 tbsp (35 g)	40	1	23	.5	11	0
Cheese Dip, Jalapeño & Cheddar, Frito-Lay's 2 tbsp (34 g)	50	3	54	1	18	5

FOOD/PORTION SIZE	CAL	FAT Total (g)	FAT As % of Cal	SAT FAT Total (g)	SAT FAT As % of Cal	CHOL (mg)
Cheese Dip, Mild Cheddar, Frito-Lay's, 2 tbsp (34 g)	50	3	54	1	18	5
Dill, Deans, 2 tbsp (31 g)	60	5	75	1	15	0
French Onion, Deans, 2 tbsp (31 g)	60	5	75	1	15	0
French Onion, Light, Deans, 2 tbsp (31 g)	35	2	51	1	26	10
French Onion, No Fat, Deans, 2 tbsp (31 g)	30	0	0	0	0	<5
French Onion, Ruffles Dip, 2 tbsp (33 g)	70	5	64	1	13	0
French Onion, with Bacon, Deans, 2 tbsp (31 g)	60	5	75	1	15	0
Ranch, Deans, 2 tbsp (31 g)	60	5	75	1	15	0
Ranch, No Fat, Deans, 2 tbsp (31 g)	30	0	0	0	0	<5
Ranch, Ruffles Dip, 2 tbsp (33 g)	70	6	77	1	13	0
Salsa, Jays, 2 tbsp (30 g)	15	0	0	0	0	0
Veggie, No Fat, Deans, 2 tbsp (31 g)	30	0	0	0	0	<5

FRUIT SNACKS

Apple Cinnamon, Frosted, Pop-Tarts, Low Fat, Kellogg's, 1 pastry (52 g)	190	3	14	.5	2	0
Blueberry, Frosted, Pop-Tarts, Kellogg's, 1 pastry (52 g)	200	5	23	1	5	0
Cherry, Frosted, Pop-Tarts, Kellogg's, 1 pastry (52 g)	200	5	23	1	5	0
Cherry Fruit Roll-Ups, Betty Crocker, 2 rolls (28 g)	110	1	8	0	0	0
Strawberry, Frosted, Pop-Tarts, Kellogg's, 1 pastry (52 g)	200	5	3	1.5	7	0
Strawberry, Fruit Roll-Ups, Betty Crocker, 2 rolls (28 g)	110	1	8	.5	4	na

SNACKS

FOOD/PORTION SIZE	CAL	FAT Total (g)	FAT As % of Cal	SAT FAT Total (g)	SAT FAT As % of Cal	CHOL (mg)
GRANOLA						
Apple Berry, Granola Bar, Quaker, 1 bar (28 g)	110	2	16	.5	4	0
ChipsAhoy!, Granola Bar, Nabisco, 1 bar (28 g)	120	4	30	1	8	0
Oatmeal Cookie, Granola Bar, Quaker, 1 bar (28 g)	110	2	16	.5	4	0
Oreo, Granola Bar, Nabisco, 1 bar (28 g)	120	4	30	1	8	0
Peanut Butter Chocolate Chip, Chewy Granola Bar, Quaker Oats, 1 bar (28 g)	120	<5	<34	<2	<11	0
S'mores, Granola Bar, Quaker, 1 bar (28 g)	110	2	16	.5	4	0
POPCORN						
Air-popped, unsalted, 1 cup	30	tr	na	tr	na	0
Caramel Corn, Buttery Toffee, Fat-Free, Louise's, 1 cup (28 g)	100	0	0	0	0	0
Caramel Corn, Fat Free, Louise's, 7/8 cup (28 g)	100	0	0	0	0	0
Microwave, Butter, Light, Orville Redenbacher's, unpopped, 2 tbsp (33 g)	120	6	45	1	8	0
Microwave, Original Butter, Pop Secret, unpopped, 2 tbsp (34 g)	170	13	69	2.5	13	0
Pop-Air-Popped, Unsalted, Original, Orville Redenbacher's, popped, 1cup	15	0	0	0	0	na
Popped, O-Ke-Doke, Buttery, Jays, popped in vegetable oil, 3 cups (28 g)	150	10	60	2	12	0

FOOD/PORTION SIZE	CAL	FAT Total (g)	FAT As % of Cal	SAT FAT Total (g)	SAT FAT As % of Cal	CHOL (mg)
Popped in vegetable oil, salted, 1 cup	55	3	49	<1	<8	0
Sugar syrup coated, 1 cup	135	1	6	<1	<1	0
POTATO CHIPS						
Jays, Curly Dippettes, 15 chips (28 g)	150	10	60	1.5	9	0
Lays, 20 chips (28 g)	150	10	60	3	18	0
Lays, Hickory Bar-B-Que, about 15 chips (28 g)	150	10	60	2	12	0
Pringles, Original, 14 chips (28 g)	160	11	62	3	17	0
Pringles, Light Crisps, Ranch, (⅓ less fat than regular Pringles) 16 chips (28 g)	140	7	45	2	13	0
Pringles, Sour Cream n' Onion, about 14 crisps (28 g)	160	10	56	<3	<17	0
Ruffles, 17 chips (28 g)	160	10	56	3	17	0
Ruffles, Reduced Fat, (⅓ less fat than regular Ruffles) 16 chips (28 g)	140	6.7	43	1	6	0
PRETZELS						
Pretzel Chips, Mr. Phipps, 16 chips, 1 oz (28 g)	100	0	0	0	0	0
Rods, Rold Gold, 3 pretzels (28 g)	110	1.5	12	.5	4	0
Sticks, Fat Free, Rold Gold, 48 pretzels (28 g)	110	0	0	0	0	0
Twisted Dutch, Anderson, 2 pretzels (32 g)	130	1	7	0	0	0
Twisted Thin, Fat Free, Rold Gold, 12 pretzels (28 g)	110	0	0	0	0	0
Twisted Thin, Jays, 13 pretzels (30 g)	110	0	0	0	0	0

Soups

FOOD/PORTION SIZE	CAL	FAT Total (g)	FAT As % of Cal	SAT FAT Total (g)	SAT FAT As % of Cal	CHOL (mg)
Asparagus, Cream of, Campbell's, 4 oz condensed, 8 oz as prepared, 1 cup (120 ml)	110	7	57	2	16	5
Bean, Salsa, Home Cookin', Campbell's, 1 cup (240 ml)	190	1	5	.5	2	0
Bean 'n' Ham, Chunky Soup, Ready to Serve, Campbell's, 1 cup (240 ml)	190	2	9	.5	2	15
Bean with Bacon, Campbell's, condensed, ½ cup (120 ml)	180	5	25	2	10	<5
Beef Broth, Ready to Serve, Swanson 1 cup (240 ml)	20	1	45	.5	2	15
Beef broth bouillon consommé, canned, condensed, prepared with water, 1 cup	29	0	0	0	0	0
Beef Noodle, Campbell's, condensed, ½ cup (120 ml)	70	2.5	32	1	13	15
Bouillon, Chicken, Wylers, 1 cube	5	0	0	0	0	0
Broccoli Cheese & Rice, Hearty Soup, Uncle Ben's, 1 cup cooked	160	3	17	1.5	8	5
Chicken, Cream of, Campbell's, condensed, ½ cup (120 ml)	130	8	55	3	21	10
Chicken, Cream of, with Vegetables, Healthy Choice, 1 cup (254 g)	130	2	14	1	7	10
Chicken Mushroom Chowder, Chunky, Campbell's, 1 cup (240 ml)	210	12	51	4	17	10

FOOD/PORTION SIZE	CAL	FAT Total (g)	FAT As % of Cal	SAT FAT Total (g)	SAT FAT As % of Cal	CHOL (mg)
Chicken Noodle, Campbell's, condensed, ½ cup (120 ml)	60	2	30	1	15	15
Chicken Noodle, Dehydrated, Soup Secrets, Lipton, 3 tbsp, 8 fluid oz prepared	80	2.5	28	1	11	15
Chicken Noodle, Hearty, Healthy Request, Campbell's, 1 cup (120 ml)	160	3	17	1	12	20
Chicken Noodle, Lipton Cup-a-Soup, 1 envelope, 6 fluid oz prepared	50	1	18	0	0	0
Chicken Noodle, Old Fashioned, Healthy Choice, 1 cup (250 g)	140	3	19	1	6	10
Chicken Noodle, Progresso, 1 cup (238 g)	80	1.5	17	.5	6	25
Chicken Rice, Campbell's, condensed, ½ cup (120 ml)	70	2.5	32	1	13	<5
Clam Chowder, New England, Ready to Serve, Healthy Choice, 1 cup (251 g)	120	1.5	11	1	8	10
Minestrone, Home Cookin', Campbell's, 1 cup (240 ml)	120	2	15	1	8	5
Minestrone, Original Recipe, Progresso, 1 cup (240 g)	130	2.5	17	.5	3	0
Mushroom, Cream of, Campbell's, condensed, ½ cup (120 ml)	110	7	57	2.5	20	<5
Mushroom, Cream of, Healthy Request, Campbell's, condensed, ½ cup (120 ml)	70	3	39	1	13	10
Onion, Dehydrated, Recipe Secrets, Lipton, 1 tbsp, 1 cup prepared	20	0	0	0	0	0

SOUPS

FOOD/PORTION SIZE	CAL	FAT Total (g)	FAT As % of Cal	SAT FAT Total (g)	SAT FAT As % of Cal	CHOL (mg)
Pea, Green, Campbell's, condensed, ½ cup (120 ml)	180	3	15	1	5	<5
Pea, Split, with Ham and Bacon, Campbell's, condensed, ½ cup (120 ml)	180	3.5	18	2	10	<5
Tomato, Campbell's, condensed, ½ cup (120 ml)	100	2	18	0	0	0
Tomato vegetable, dehydrated, prepared with water, 6 oz	40	1	23	<1	<7	0
Turkey Noodle, Campbell's, condensed, ½ cup (120 ml)	80	<3	28	1	11	15
Vegetable, Vegetarian, Campbell's, condensed, ½ cup (120 ml)	70	1	13	0	0	0
Vegetable Beef, Campbell's, condensed, ½ cup (120 ml)	80	2	23	1	11	10
Vegetable Beef, Healthy Request, Campbell's, ½ cup (120 ml)	80	2	23	1	11	5

Vegetables

FOOD/PORTION SIZE	CAL	FAT Total (g)	FAT As % of Cal	SAT FAT Total (g)	SAT FAT As % of Cal	CHOL (mg)
ALFALFA						
Seeds, sprouted, raw, 1 cup	10	tr	na	tr	na	0
ARTICHOKES						
Globe or French, cooked, drained, 1 artichoke	53	tr	na	tr	na	0

FOOD/PORTION SIZE	CAL	FAT Total (g)	FAT As % of Cal	SAT FAT Total (g)	SAT FAT As % of Cal	CHOL (mg)
Hearts, Canned, Reese, 2 pieces with liquid	50	0	0	0	0	0
Jerusalem, red, sliced, 1 cup	114	tr	na	0	0	0
ASPARAGUS						
Cuts, Raw, Birds Eye, ½ cup (95 g)	25	0	0	0	0	0
Cuts & tips, cooked, drained, raw, 1 cup	45	1	20	<1	<2	0
Cuts & tips, frozen, 1 cup	50	1	18	<1	<4	0
Spears, Canned, Cut, Green Giant, ½ cup	20	0	0	0	0	0
Spears, Canned, Extra Long, Green Giant, 5 spears, 4.5 oz	20	0	0	0	0	0
Spears, raw, cooked, drained, 4 spears	15	tr	na	tr	na	0
Spears, Frozen, Birds Eye, 8 spears	20	0	0	0	0	0
BAMBOO SHOOTS						
Canned, drained, 1 cup	25	1	36	<1	<4	0
Canned, Sliced, LaChoy, ½ cup (114 g)	25	0	0	0	0	0
BEANS						
Green, Cut, Canned, Green Giant, ½ cup (120 g)	20	0	0	0	0	0
Green, Cut, Frozen, Birds Eye, ½ cup (83 g)	25	0	0	0	0	0
Green, French, with Toasted Almonds, Frozen, Birds Eye, 1 cup (171 g)	190	11	52	4	19	15
Green, French Cut, Birds Eye, ½ cup (83 g)	25	0	0	0	0	0
Green, French Style, Canned, Del Monte, ½ cup (121 g)	20	0	0	0	0	0

VEGETABLES

FOOD/PORTION SIZE	CAL	FAT Total (g)	FAT As % of Cal	SAT FAT Total (g)	SAT FAT As % of Cal	CHOL (mg)
Green, Italian, Canned, Del Monte, ½ cup (121 g)	30	0	0	0	0	0
Lima, Green, Canned, Del Monte, ½ cup (126 g)	80	0	0	0	0	0
Sprouts, Canned, LaChoy, 1 cup (83 g)	10	0	0	0	0	0
Sprouts (mung), cooked, drained, 1 cup	25	tr	na	tr	na	0
BEETS						
Canned, drained, solids, diced or sliced, 1 cup	55	tr	na	tr	na	0
Cooked, drained, diced or sliced, 1 cup	55	tr	na	tr	na	0
Cooked, drained, whole, 2 beets	30	tr	na	tr	na	0
Greens, leaves and stems, cooked, drained, 1 cup	40	tr	na	tr	na	0
Pickled, Ruby Red, Bottled, Whole, Aunt Nellie's, 2 beets (36 g)	25	0	0	0	0	0
Ruby Red, Sliced, Bottled, Aunt Nellie's, ½ cup (120 g)	40	0	0	0	0	0
BROCCOLI						
Chopped, Birds Eye, ⅓ cup (86 g)	25	0	0	0	0	0
Chopped, frozen, cooked, drained, 1 cup	50	tr	na	tr	na	0
Frozen, cooked, drained, 1 piece (4½–5 in. long)	10	tr	na	tr	na	0
Raw, 1 spear	40	1	23	<1	<2	0
Spears, raw, cooked, drained, 1 cup (½-in. pieces)	45	tr	na	<1	<2	0

FOOD/PORTION SIZE	CAL	FAT Total (g)	FAT As % of Cal	SAT FAT Total (g)	SAT FAT As % of Cal	CHOL (mg)
Spears, Select, Green Giant, 3 spears, 3 oz	25	0	0	0	0	0
BRUSSELS SPROUTS						
Baby, in Butter Sauce, Green Giant, ⅔ cup (104 g)	60	1.5	23	1.5	23	<5
Frozen, cooked, drained, 1 cup	65	1	14	<1	<1	0
Raw, cooked, drained, 1 cup	60	1	15	<1	<3	0
CABBAGE						
Chinese pak-choi, cooked, drained, 1 cup	20	tr	na	tr	na	0
Chinese pe-tsai, raw, 1 cup (1-in. pieces)	10	tr	na	tr	na	0
Common varieties, cooked, drained, 1 cup	30	tr	na	tr	na	0
Red, raw, coarsely shredded or sliced, 1 cup	20	tr	na	tr	na	0
Savoy, raw, coarsely shredded or sliced, 1 cup	20	tr	na	tr	na	0
CARROTS						
Baby, Cut, Harvest Fresh, Green Giant, ⅔ cup, ½ cup cooked	20	0	0	0	0	0
Canned, Sliced, Del Monte, ½ cup (123 g)	35	0	0	0	0	0
Frozen, sliced, cooked, drained, 1 cup	55	tr	na	tr	na	0
Raw, sliced, cooked, drained, 1 cup	70	tr	na	<1	<1	0
Raw, w/o crowns or tips, scraped, grated, 1 cup	45	tr	na	tr	na	0

VEGETABLES

FOOD/PORTION SIZE	CAL	FAT Total (g)	FAT As % of Cal	SAT FAT Total (g)	SAT FAT As % of Cal	CHOL (mg)
CAULIFLOWER						
Florets, Frozen, Green Giant, 1 cup frozen, ⅔ cup cooked	25	0	0	0	0	0
Flowerets, frozen, cooked, drained, 1 cup	35	tr	na	<1	<3	0
Flowerets, raw, cooked, drained, 1 cup	30	tr	na	tr	na	0
CELERY						
Pascal type, raw, large outer stalk, 1 stalk	5	tr	na	tr	na	0
Pascal type, raw, pieces, diced, 1 cup	20	tr	na	tr	na	0
COLLARDS						
Frozen, chopped, cooked, drained, 1 cup	60	1	15	<1	<2	0
Raw, leaves w/o stems, cooked, drained, 1 cup	25	tr	na	<1	<4	0
CORN						
Niblets, Frozen, Green Giant, ⅔ cup frozen, ½ cup cooked	80	.5	6	0	0	0
Niblets, in Butter Sauce, Frozen, Green Giant, ⅔ cup	130	3	21	1.5	10	<5
Shoepeg, White, Harvest Fresh, Green Giant, ½ cup	70	.5	6	0	0	0
Sweet, Cream Style, Canned, Green Giant, ½ cup (120 g)	100	.5	5	0	0	0
Sweet, frozen, cooked, drained, 1 ear (3½ in.)	60	tr	na	<1	<2	0

FOOD/PORTION SIZE	CAL	FAT Total (g)	FAT As % of Cal	SAT FAT Total (g)	SAT FAT As % of Cal	CHOL (mg)
Sweet, kernels, cooked, drained, 1 cup	135	tr	na	tr	na	0
Sweet, on the Cob, Frozen, Birds Eye, 2 ears	110	1	8	0	0	0
Sweet, raw, cooked, drained, 1 ear (5 x 1¾ in.)	85	1	11	<1	<2	0
Sweet, whole kernel, vacuum packed, 1 cup	165	1	5	<1	<1	0
Whole Kernel, Canned, Del Monte, ½ cup (125 g)	90	1	10	0	0	0
Whole Kernel, No Salt Added, Canned, Del Monte, ½ cup (125 g)	60	1	15	0	0	0
CUCUMBER						
Peeled slices, ⅛-in. thick (large 2⅛-in. diameter, small 1¾-in. diameter), 6 large or 8 small	5	tr	na	tr	na	0
EGGPLANT						
Cooked, steamed, 1 cup	25	tr	na	tr	na	0
ENDIVE						
Curly (including escarole), raw, small pieces, 1 cup	10	tr	na	tr	na	0
GREENS						
Dandelion, cooked, drained, 1 cup	34	1	26	<1	<3	0
Mustard, Canned, The Allens, ½ cup (118 g)	30	.5	15	0	0	0
Mustard, w/o stems and midribs, cooked, drained, 1 cup	20	tr	na	tr	na	0
Turnip, Canned, The Allens, ½ cup (121 g)	25	.5	18	0	0	0

VEGETABLES

FOOD/PORTION SIZE	CAL	FAT Total (g)	FAT As % of Cal	SAT FAT Total (g)	SAT FAT As % of Cal	CHOL (mg)
Turnip, Chopped, Frozen, Seabrook Farms, 3.3 oz	20	0	0	0	0	0
Turnip, frozen, chopped, cooked, drained, 1 cup	50	1	19	<1	<4	0
Turnip, raw, leaves & stems, cooked, drained, 1 cup	30	tr	na	<1	<3	0
KALE						
Frozen, chopped, cooked, drained, 1 cup	40	1	23	<1	<2	0
Raw, chopped, cooked, drained, 1 cup	40	1	23	<1	<2	0
KOHLRABI						
Thickened bulblike stem, cooked, drained, diced, 1 cup	50	tr	na	tr	na	0
LETTUCE						
Butterhead, as Boston types, raw, leaves, 1 outer leaf or 2 inner leaves	tr	tr	na	tr	na	0
Crisphead, as iceberg, raw, ¼ of head, 1 wedge	20	tr	na	tr	na	0
Crisphead, as iceberg, raw, pieces, chopped, shredded, 1 cup	5	tr	na	tr	na	0
Looseleaf (bunching varieties including romaine or cos), chopped or shredded, 1 cup	10	tr	na	tr	na	0
MIXED VEGETABLES						
Bavarian Green Beans Spaetzle, Birds Eye International Recipe, 1 cup (151 g)	160	8	45	<5	<25	50

FOOD/PORTION SIZE	CAL	FAT		SAT FAT		CHOL (mg)
		Total (g)	As % of Cal	Total (g)	As % of Cal	
Broccoli, Baby Carrots, Water Chestnuts, Farm Fresh Mix, Birds Eye, ½ cup (95 g)	30	0	0	0	0	0
Broccoli, Cauliflower, Carrots, Farm Fresh Mix, Birds Eye, ½ cup (92 g)	25	0	0	0	0	0
Broccoli, Red Pepper, Onion & Mushrooms, Farm Fresh Mix, Birds Eye, ½ cup	25	0	0	0	0	0
Cauliflower in Cheese Sauce, Green Giant, ½ cup	60	<3	<38	<1	<8	<5
French Green Beans, with Toasted Almonds, Bird's Eye, 1 cup (171 g)	190	11	52	4	19	15
Japanese Style, International Recipe, Birds Eye, ½ cup (127 g)	80	<5	<51	3	34	10
Japanese Style Vegetables, Stir Fry, International Recipe, Birds Eye, ½ cup (116 g)	35	0	0	0	0	0
New England Style Vegetables, International Recipe, Birds Eye, 1 cup	190	11	52	4	19	15
Peas, Carrots, Corn, Beans, Green Giant, ¾ cup frozen, ½ cup cooked	60	0	0	0	0	0
Rice & Broccoli, in Cheese Sauce, Green Giant, 1 container	320	12	34	4	11	15
Spinach, Creamed, Green Giant, ½ cup	80	3	34	<2	<17	0

VEGETABLES

FOOD/PORTION SIZE	CAL.	FAT Total (g)	FAT As % of Cal.	SAT. FAT Total (g)	SAT. FAT As % of Cal.	CHOL. (mg)
MUSHROOMS						
Cooked, drained, 1 cup	40	1	23	<1	<2	0
Raw, sliced or chopped, 1 cup	20	tr	na	tr	na	0
Sliced, Bottled, Green Giant, ½ cup with liquid (120 g)	30	0	0	0	0	0
Sliced, Bottled, No Salt Added, Pennsylvania Dutchman, ½ cup with liquid (130 g)	20	0	0	0	0	0
Solids, canned, drained, 1 cup	35	tr	na	<1	<3	0
Stems & Pieces, Canned, Pennsylvania Dutchman, ½ cup with liquid (130 g)	20	0	0	0	0	0
OKRA						
Pods, 3 x ⅝ in., cooked, 8 pods	27	tr	na	tr	na	0
Pods, Whole, Frozen, Pict Sweet, 9 pods	25	0	0	0	0	0
ONIONS						
Holland-Style, Whole, Aunt Nellies, ½ cup (122 g)	40	0	0	0	0	0
Raw, chopped, 1 cup	55	tr	na	<1	<2	0
Raw, sliced, 1 cup	40	tr	na	<1	<2	0
Rings, Frozen, Ore Ida, 6 rings	230	13	51	2.5	10	0
Spring, raw, bulb (⅜-in. diameter) and white portion of top, 6 onions	10	tr	na	tr	na	0
Whole or sliced, cooked, drained, 1 cup	60	tr	na	<1	<2	0

FOOD/PORTION SIZE	CAL	FAT Total (g)	FAT As % of Cal	SAT FAT Total (g)	SAT FAT As % of Cal	CHOL (mg)
PARSLEY						
Freeze-dried, 1 tbsp	tr	tr	tr	tr	tr	0
Raw, 10 sprigs	5	tr	na	tr	na	0
PARSNIPS						
Diced or 2-in. lengths, cooked, drained, 1 cup	125	tr	na	<1	<1	0
PEAS						
Black-Eyed, Canned, The Allens, ½ cup (126 g)	120	1	8	.5	4	0
Blackeye, Frozen, Pict Sweet, ½ cup (81 g)	110	1	8	0	0	0
Black-eyed, raw, immature seeds, cooked, drained, 1 cup	180	1	5	<1	<2	0
Green, Baby, Early, Frozen, Harvest Fresh, Green Giant, ⅔ cup frozen, ½ cup cooked	70	0	0	0	0	0
Green, solids, canned, drained, 1 cup	115	1	8	<1	<1	0
Pods, edible, cooked, drained, 1 cup	65	tr	na	<1	<1	0
Sweet, Canned, Green Giant, ½ cup (122 g)	60	0	0	0	0	0
Sweet, Very Young, Small, Canned, Del Monte, ½ cup (125 g)	60	0	0	0	0	0
PEPPERS						
Cherry, Mild, Bottled, Vlasic, 2 peppers, 1 oz	10	0	0	0	0	0
Hot chili, raw, 1 pepper	20	tr	na	tr	na	0
Jalapeño, Hot, Bottled, Vlasic, ¼ cup drained	10	0	0	0	0	0

VEGETABLES

FOOD/PORTION SIZE	CAL	FAT Total (g)	FAT As % of Cal	SAT FAT Total (g)	SAT FAT As % of Cal	CHOL (mg)
Mexican, Tiny, Hot, Bottled, Vlasic, 9 peppers, 1 oz	10	0	0	0	0	0
Pepperoncini, Bottled, Vlasic, 2 peppers, 1 oz	5	0	0	0	0	0
Sweet (about 5 per lb, whole), stem and seeds removed, 1 pepper	20	tr	na	tr	na	0
Sweet (about 5 per lb, whole), stem and seeds removed, cooked, drained, 1 pepper	15	tr	na	tr	na	0

PICKLES

FOOD/PORTION SIZE	CAL	FAT Total (g)	FAT As % of Cal	SAT FAT Total (g)	SAT FAT As % of Cal	CHOL (mg)
Bread & Butter Chips, Zesty, Bottled, Vlasic, 10 chips, 1 oz	45	0	0	0	0	0
Cucumber, dill, medium whole (3¾-in. long, 1¼-in. diameter), 1 pickle	5	tr	na	tr	na	0
Cucumber, fresh-pack slices, (1½-in. diameter, ¼-in. thick), 2 slices	10	tr	na	tr	na	0
Cucumber, sweet gherkin, small, (whole, about 2½-in. long, ¾-in. diameter), 1 pickle	20	tr	na	tr	na	0
Dill, Spears, Kosher, Bottled, Vlasic, 1 spear, 1 oz	5	0	0	0	0	0
Dill, Whole, Crunchy, Kosher, Bottled, Vlasic, ½ pickle, 1 oz	5	0	0	0	0	0
Gherkins, Sweet, Bottled, Vlasic, 3 pickles, 1 oz	40	0	0	0	0	0
Hamburger, Dill Chips, Original, Bottled, Vlasic, 10 chips, 1 oz	5	0	0	0	0	0
Midgets, Tiny, Sweet, Bottled, Vlasic, 4 pickles, 1 oz	40	0	0	0	0	0

FOOD/PORTION SIZE	CAL	FAT Total (g)	FAT As % of Cal	SAT FAT Total (g)	SAT FAT As % of Cal	CHOL (mg)
POTATOES						
Baked (about 2 per lb. raw), flesh only, 1 potato	145	tr	na	tr	na	0
Baked (about 2 per lb. raw), with skin, 1 potato	220	tr	na	<1	<1	0
Boiled (about 3 per lb. raw), peeled before boiling, 1 potato	115	tr	na	tr	na	0
French fried strip (2 to 3½ in. long), fried in vegetable oil, 10 strips	160	8	45	3	17	0
French fried strip (2 to 3½ in. long), oven heated, 10 strips	110	4	33	2	16	0
French Fries, Microwave Ready, Snakin' Fries, Frozen, Ore Ida, 1 pkg, 5 oz (151 g)	340	20	53	3.5	9	0
French Fries, Frozen, Ore Ida, 16 fries	120	4	30	.5	4	0
Red, raw, 1 potato, 5.5 oz (148 g)	120	0	0	0	0	0
Sweet, candied, 2½ x 2-in. piece, 1 piece	145	3	19	1	6	8
Sweet, cooked (baked in skin), 1 potato	115	tr	na	tr	na	0
Sweet, cooked (boiled w/o skin), 1 potato	160	tr	na	<1	<1	0
Sweet, Cut Yams, Canned, Princella, ⅔ cup (166 g)	160	.5	3	0	0	0
Sweet, Frozen, Ore Ida, 5 pieces with sauce	190	0	0	0	0	0
Sweet, vacuum pack, 2¾ x 1-in. piece	35	tr	na	tr	na	0
Tater Tots, Ore Ida, 9 pieces (85 g)	160	8	45	1.5	8	0

VEGETABLES

FOOD/PORTION SIZE	CAL	FAT Total (g)	FAT As % of Cal	SAT FAT Total (g)	SAT FAT As % of Cal	CHOL (mg)
Twice Baked, Butter Flavor, Ore Ida, 1 piece (141 g)	170	6	32	1	5	0
Wedges, Texas Crispers, Ore Ida, 3 oz, 7 wedges	150	7	42	1	6	0
Whole, New, Canned, Del Monte, 2 medium	60	0	0	0	0	0
PUMPKIN						
Canned, 1 cup	85	1	11	<1	<4	0
Pie Mix, Libby's, ½ cup (106 g)	100	0	0	0	0	0
Raw, Cooked, mashed, 1 cup	50	tr	na	<1	<2	0
Solid Pack, 100% Natural, Libby's, ½ cup (122 g)	40	.5	11	na	na	na
RADISHES						
Raw, stem ends and rootlets cut off, 4 radishes	5	tr	na	tr	na	0
SPINACH						
Harvest Fresh, Green Giant, ½ cup (100 g)	25	0	0	0	0	0
Leaf, frozen, cooked, drained, 1 cup	55	tr	na	<1	<2	0
Raw, chopped, 1 cup	10	tr	na	tr	na	0
Raw, cooked, drained, 1 cup	40	tr	na	<1	<2	0
Whole Leaf, Canned, Del Monte, ½ cup (115 g)	30	0	0	0	0	0
SQUASH						
Summer (all varieties), cooked, sliced, drained, 1 cup	35	1	26	<1	<3	0

FOOD/PORTION SIZE	CAL	FAT		SAT FAT		CHOL (mg)
		Total (g)	As % of Cal	Total (g)	As % of Cal	
TOMATOES						
Juice, Bottled, Campbell's, 8 fluid oz (240 ml)	50	0	0	0	0	0
Juice, canned, 1 cup	40	tr	na	tr	na	0
Paste, canned, 1 cup	220	2	8	<1	<1	0
Paste, Canned, Contadina, 2 tbsp (33 g)	30	0	0	0	0	0
Paste, Italian, 2 tbsp (33 g)	30	.5	15	0	0	0
Puree, canned, 1 cup	105	tr	na	tr	na	0
Puree, Canned, Contadina, ¼ cup (63 g)	20	0	0	0	0	0
Raw, 2³/₅-in. diameter (3 per 12-oz pkg), 1 tomato	25	tr	na	tr	na	0
Sauce, Extra Thick & Zesty, Canned, Contadina, ¼ cup (61 g)	20	0	0	0	0	0
Sauce, Italian Style, Canned, Contadina, ¼ cup (61 g)	15	0	0	0	0	0
Sauce, Pasta Ready, Canned, Contadina, ½ cup (122 g)	40	1.5	34	0	0	0
Stewed, Canned, Hunts, ½ cup (121 g)	35	0	0	0	0	0
Stewed, Italian Style, Canned, Contadina, ½ cup (122 g)	40	0	0	0	0	0
Stewed, Mexican Recipe, Canned, Del Monte, ½ cup (126 g)	35	0	0	0	0	0
VEGETABLES WITH SAUCE						
Broccoli with Cheese Sauce, Birds Eye Cheese Sauce Combination Vegetables, ½ cup (127 g)	70	3	39	<2	<19	10
Brussels Sprouts in Butter Sauce, Green Giant, ⅔ cup (104 g)	60	1.5	23	1.5	23	<5

VEGETABLES

FOOD/PORTION SIZE	CAL	FAT Total (g)	FAT As % of Cal	SAT FAT Total (g)	SAT FAT As % of Cal	CHOL (mg)
Cauliflower with Cheese Flavored Sauce, Green Giant, ½ cup (99 g)	60	<3	<38	<1	<8	<5
Italian Style Vegetables, Birds Eye International Recipe, 1 cup (159 g)	140	9	58	<4	<23	15

Yogurt

FOOD/PORTION SIZE	CAL	FAT Total (g)	FAT As % of Cal	SAT FAT Total (g)	SAT FAT As % of Cal	CHOL (mg)
Blueberry, Dannon, 1 container (227 g)	240	3	11	<2	<6	15
Blueberry, Light 'n Lively, 1 container	140	1	6	<1	<3	10
Cheesecake, Double Delights, Dannon, 1 container (170 g)	170	1	5	.5	3	10
Cherry, Original, Yoplait, 1 container (170 g)	180	1.5	8	1	5	10
Plain, Premium, Dannon, 1 container (227 g)	140	4	26	2	13	20
Raspberry, Fat Free, Yoplait, 1 container (170 g)	160	0	0	0	0	5
Strawberry, Light, Nonfat, Dannon, 1 container (125 g)	60	0	0	0	0	0
Strawberry, Original, Yoplait, 1 container (170 g)	170	<2	<8	1	5	10
Trix, Triple Cherry, Yoplait, 1 container (170 g)	160	2	11	1	6	5
Vanilla, Frozen, Edy's, ½ cup (65 g)	100	2.5	23	1.5	14	10
Vanilla, with Chocolate Crunchies, Light 'N Crunchy, Dannon, 1 container (227 g)	150	0	0	0	0	<5